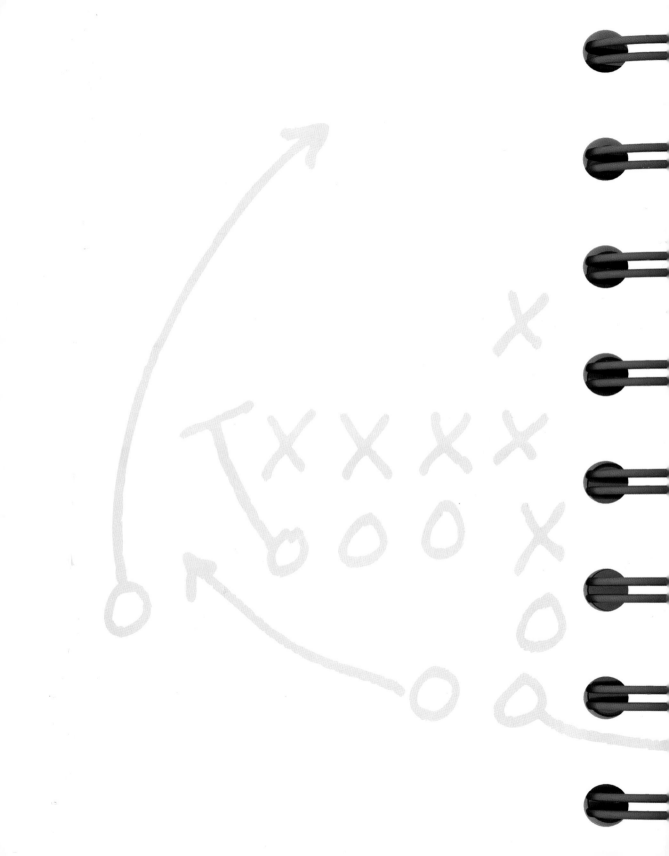

Sacking Obesity

Sacking Obesity

The Team Tiger Game Plan for Kids
Who Want to Lose Weight, Feel Great, and
Win on and off the Playing Field

Tiger Greene

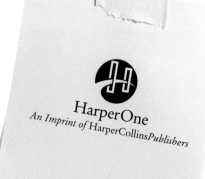

HarperOne
An Imprint of HarperCollinsPublishers

This book is written as a source of information only. The information contained in this book should by no means be considered a substitute for the advice of a qualified medical professional, who should always be consulted before you begin any new diet, exercise, or other health program.

All efforts have been made to ensure the accuracy of the information contained in this book as of the date published. The publisher and the author disclaim liability for any adverse effects that may occur as a result of applying the methods suggested in this book.

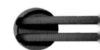

HarperCollins books may be purchased for educational, business, or sales promotional use. For information, please e-mail the Special Markets Department at SPsales@harpercollins.com.

HarperCollins website: http://www.harpercollins.com

HarperCollins®, 📖®, and HarperOne™ are trademarks of HarperCollins Publishers.

Book design by Ralph Fowler / rlfdesign

FIRST EDITION

Library of Congress Cataloging-in-Publication Data
Greene, Tiger.
    Sacking obesity : the Team Tiger game plan for kids who want to lose weight, feel great, and win on and off the playing field / by Tiger Greene. —First edition.
        pages   cm
    ISBN 978-0-06-213575-9
    1. Greene, Tiger—Health.   2. Obesity in children.   3. Physical fitness.
I. Title.
    RJ399.C6G755   2012
    618.92'398—dc23   2012010707

12 13 14 15 16   RRD(H)   10 9 8 7 6 5 4 3 2 1

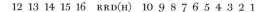

This book is dedicated to the Team Tiger Ohana. The Team Tiger Ohana is a family. It consists of everybody who has helped me continue and go forward with my journey. From all the experts at our camps, the volunteers, the campers, Coach Z and his family, and of course my family. Zack, Kaila, Michael, my mom, my dad, all of my uncles and aunts and grandmas and grandpas. All of the people listed here have given me so much support not only at the start of my journey, but to pursue it into what it is today. Thank you so much everyone. I love you all so much for your support and encouragement.

Ohana forever . . .

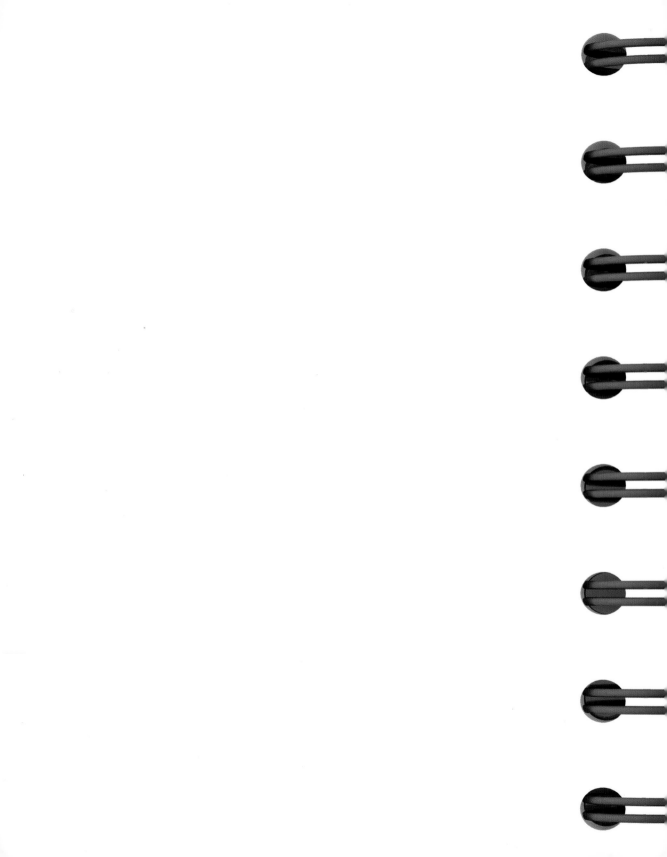

Contents

Part 1: **My Journey**

1. Tunnel Vision   3

2. Family, Football, Food . . .
   and the Decision to Change   27

Part 2: **Follow Me Into . . .
Eating Healthy**

3. What's Up, Doc?   51
   EDUCATION STATION 1

4. Checkup from the Neck Up   71
   EDUCATION STATION 2

5. Eat like a Tiger!   89
   EDUCATION STATION 3

6. Eating Out: It's All About Choices   113
   EDUCATION STATION 4

Part 3: Follow Me Into . . . An Active Life

7. Agility   137

ACTIVITY STATION 1

8. Quickness   159

ACTIVITY STATION 2

9. Strength   175

ACTIVITY STATION 3

10. Flexibility   191

ACTIVITY STATION 4

Epilogue   209

About Tiger Greene   217

Acknowledgments   219

Index   221

PART 1

My Journey

When you look up *journey* in the dictionary, you find this definition: "the act of traveling from one place to another." Between December 8, 2009, and now, I've traveled pretty far from where I started. I guess you could say I've traveled from sickness to health, shyness to self-confidence, follower to leader. I also lost a lot of weight, which is cool, but what's even cooler is that, by taking this journey, I found out who I am.

I wrote this book to help *you* get started on *your* journey. You can take that first step anytime you want. But before you go, you need to know where you're starting from and where you want to go. To see the path I traveled, turn the page . . .

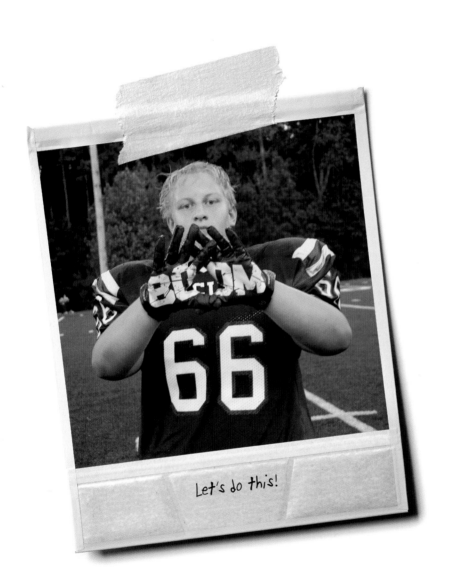

Let's do this!

CHAPTER 1

Tunnel Vision

It's a cool Saturday morning in April, but they say it's always sunny and seventy in the Georgia Dome, and that's where I am: in the tunnel with NFL great Marcus Stroud and five other NFL players—Brian Finneran and Mike Peterson of the Falcons, Drayton Florence of the Buffalo Bills, Byron Leftwich of the Pittsburgh Steelers, and Brian Kozlowski, a former Falcon and Redskin.

I've dreamed about this moment for so many years. About sitting in this exact tunnel with my Falcons jersey on, waiting for my name to be announced so I can take the field for my first NFL game. Well, here I am, waiting for my name to be announced. But I'm thirteen and instead of a Falcons jersey, I'm wearing a Team Tiger Sacking Obesity T-shirt.

Okay, so the moment isn't exactly the way I dreamed it. But I couldn't feel any prouder. In a few minutes, almost three hundred overweight kids and their families will begin the journey I started a little over a year ago.

Back then, I was a two-hundred-fifty-pound kid eating his way through

3

life. No self-confidence. No clear destination. Today, I'm fifty pounds lighter. I actually enjoy wearing nice clothes. I'm off all the medications I had to take for the health issues my weight had caused. I can run laps at football practice. And I just don't think about food the way I used to. I'm a kid with a mission: to help big kids all over the world turn their health and their lives around. That mission was all I lived for. It put me in this tunnel.

LOL. I have tunnel vision!

It's funny, but true. I was totally focused on changing my life and on that mission. My every waking moment was about turning my dream into a reality. Nothing was gonna stop me. Not how bad my knees hurt after those first few runs with Mom. Not those first days of eating

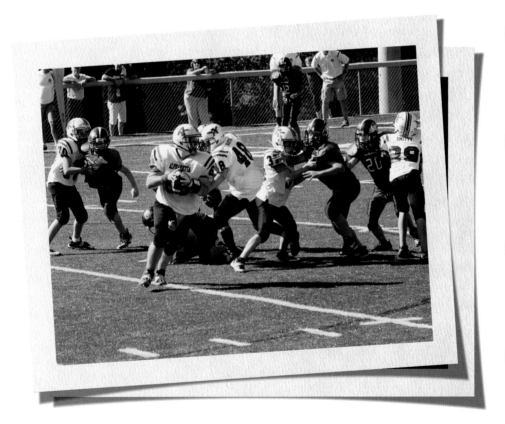

#66 The Greene Machine

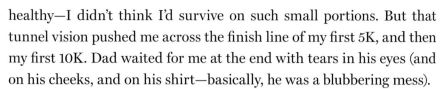

healthy—I didn't think I'd survive on such small portions. But that tunnel vision pushed me across the finish line of my first 5K, and then my first 10K. Dad waited for me at the end with tears in his eyes (and on his cheeks, and on his shirt—basically, he was a blubbering mess).

What a difference a year makes.

I look out over the field. Onstage at midfield, our master of ceremonies tests the sound system. My coach and friend Andrew Zumwalt—Coach Z to the hundreds of kids he's helped, including me—runs around like a crazy man, helping volunteers set up the stations. All over the field, the doctors and nutritionists I've met, who are here to teach and show the kids and their families how to make healthy changes, set up chairs.

But I won't give you or any of the kids who come to my camps any boring lectures about childhood obesity. Been there, done that, got the T-shirt to prove it. When you go on a journey, the trip should be fun and the food should be good. So in the end zone closest to me, Shane Thompson, my friend and founder of Shane's Rib Shack, and his group get things ready for lunch. (Healthy food from the best barbecue place in Atlanta—talk about a dream come true!)

Lines of boys and girls go out for passes thrown by our volunteers. Some make awesome catches and break out their best touchdown routines. They might be a little achy tonight, but I'm betting they'll feel more happy than sore. Today, they'll learn stuff about themselves they didn't know. Do things they didn't think they could do. Come to believe that they can do anything they set their minds to.

As they go long, the kids pass right in front of the tunnel. Some see me, and our eyes meet. There's something in their eyes; I know that look. It's that little spark of hope that this—this doctor, this diet, this workout routine—might change your life. But you're afraid to trust that spark. Afraid that, like so many times before, nothing will change. And instead of igniting passion and change, that spark will just kind of smolder.

Some kids smile as they run back down the field, and I smile and nod to let them know I get it, I get them, that's why they're here. I'm gonna ignite that spark. Together with the NFL guys, Coach Z, and the doctors and nutritionists who are here to support Team Tiger, I'll turn excuses into opportunities, fear into knowledge, and the mistakes of the past into better choices in the future. We'll start their journeys together. Today.

The kids head across the dome to the tunnel on the other side, where the visiting teams take the field against the Falcons. They form a long line that disappears into the tunnel.

Oh yeah. Dad and I planned this part of the camp just this morning. They're about to make their entrance—to take the field for real.

The emcee announces the first kid, his voice swooping across the field. A girl, maybe ten years old, charges out of the tunnel, high-fiving the line of cheering volunteers and parents. At the end, she does her best "take the field" dance. I can see her grin from sixty yards away.

I watch them all take the field, past that cheering crowd, one by one, all 287 of them. My name will be called last. I'm used to it. Until a year ago, I was always picked last in playground games. No one wanted the big kid on their team. But today, being last is a great thing. It means these kids are first. Maybe for the first time ever, they get to take center stage.

The Jumbotron, which had been showing our sponsors' video loop, goes black. The kids gather around the stage, and the volunteers set up two lines from my tunnel to midfield. Then the huge screen bursts into light—photos of Marcus and me from Team Tiger's flyer. Then, blazing on the screen, my motto, "Yes We Can—Follow Me," with my name underneath. My name, on the Georgia Dome Jumbotron. Yeah, baby!

The emcee calls our station leaders to the stage. My heart pounds. That old dream comes back: I'm about to take the field.

The voice of my very proud dad echoes through the silence of the dome: "Your hosts for the day: Tiger Greene and Marcus Stroud!"

Marcus turns to me and gives me a high five. "Here we go, li'l man," he says. He's the only person who's ever called me little, but compared to his six-foot-seven stature and three hundred pounds of pure muscle, I guess I am.

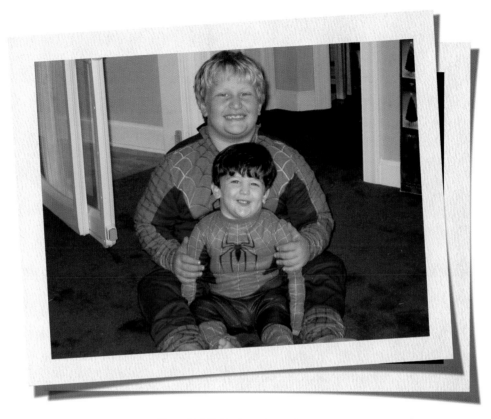

My sidekick, Zack, and me.

We run onto the field and through a wall of outstretched hands. I high-five as many as I can. We're at the thirty-yard line on the way to the stage at midfield. Something drags me down.

What's that? For some reason, I think of those fifty extra pounds I used to carry.

I look down and grin: it's my little brother, Zack, wrapped around my knees. He looks up at me, his eyes filled with pride. He's the smartest seven-year-old I know. While most kids his age used to point and make comments about my size, he always loved me—I know that. And today, he wants everyone to know I'm his big brother, running my own sports and wellness camp for other kids. Pretty awesome.

I drag Zack through the crowd and find my little sister, Kaila, who sits in front of the stage. Zack joins the family, and I step onstage with Marcus to welcome our guests.

It's game time. Time to show big kids everywhere what my motto really means.

Welcome to the Tiger Dome!

My name is Tiger Greene, I live in Alpharetta, Georgia, and as you probably know by now, I love football. From the end of July until at least Thanksgiving, my family and I are all football, all the time. I play, my dad coaches my team, Kaila is one of our cheerleaders, my mom helps as team mom, and my big brother, Mike, takes pictures and sometimes helps dad coach. Zack has started playing, and I help coach his team. So what does any of this have to do with writing a book?

I've always been the big kid. When I was six, because of my weight, I played with the eight- and nine-year-olds. That was okay—for a while. Football was the first time in my life I really felt proud, and instead of being just the big kid, I was the big, *strong* kid everyone wanted on their team. Other coaches would comment on how good I was.

But as I got older, my weight started to, well, really weigh on me. By the end of my eleven-year-old season of football—I'd just turned twelve—I weighed two hundred fifty pounds. I have always been lucky that I had really good friends and never felt alone, and I was rarely bullied to my face. But on one memorable night in 2009, my weight was no longer okay. I vowed to change my life.

With a lot of help and support from family, friends, and community, I did change my life. I call this process of getting fitter and healthier

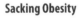

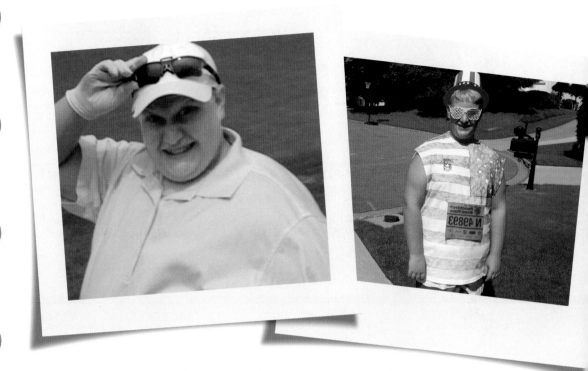

July 2009: A whole lotta Tiger to love! Here I am at the Breast Friends Golf Tournament hosted by Atlanta Falcon and friend Brian Finneran.

July 2010: Loud and proud! Right before my first 10K, the Peachtree Road Race.

my journey, and I wrote this book to help you start yours. (Check out the photos above. Some journey, right?)

Shortly after I began my journey, I started the Team Tiger Foundation. Its mission is to give big kids the education and—most of all—the support they need to help them begin their own journeys to a healthier, more active lifestyle. And because I'm a walk-the-walk type of kid, in this book, I don't ask you to eat anything or do anything that I don't do myself. So when you read about eating broccoli, just remember, it's on my plate too! This book is all about choices, changes, and how I got healthy. Most of all, it's about learning what you can do once you decide to do it, and then putting it all on the line.

Marcus and Me:
The Story of the First Team Tiger Camp

Not long after I appeared on *The Dr. Oz Show,* a friend of a friend came by the Team Tiger office and told Dad and me that she was handling publicity for a gala for Marcus Stroud, then with the Buffalo Bills. She'd seen me on the show and was very touched—her child was also fighting obesity—so she invited us to the gala to meet him.

Marcus's gala was a big ol' fancy Mardi Gras party at an Atlanta nightclub to benefit a local children's hospital. He was this monster of a man—when we shook hands, mine disappeared in his. But I felt comfortable with him right away.

On the way home, Dad and I talked about putting together an event like Marcus's to raise money for Team Tiger so we could hold a camp to help kids learn all the things I learned on my journey. During the summer of 2010, I spent most of my time writing about my journey and thinking of ways to teach kids what I learned. Near the end of that summer, one of Marcus's event coordinators, Kristie, called—she was in town and wanted to meet with us. She came to the office and asked us if we would be interested in partnering with Marcus for his next gala. In other words, Marcus would host the gala for Team Tiger.

"What would you do with your part of the funds?" she asked.

"I want to hold camps for big kids—kind of like the Super Bowl of sports camps," I said. "They'd be doing physical stuff—all the drills and exercises that Coach Z helped me do—but they'd move at their own pace. They'd have fun, because everything I do has to be fun. I'd inspire them, give them hope. And I'd get all the experts who helped me together in one place so they can help the kids like they helped me."

"It looks like we have a partnership!" my dad said.

"I have a better idea," I said. "Instead of raising money for the camp, why not just go ahead and *have* the camp?"

Dad and Kristie lit up. Now we were cooking with gas (no, not that kind of gas)!

The first thing we needed was a place to hold our camp. We narrowed it down to two options—the Georgia Dome or Georgia Tech's Bobby Dodd Stadium—and ultimately chose the dome. But the cost to rent it was more than we could swing. Dad called a friend from my youth football league, John Priore, the owner of Priority Payment Systems, a big supporter of Team Tiger.

John asked Dad how he could help, and when Dad said we needed a sponsor for the dome and the camp, he said, "You got it." It's amazing how he understood what I was trying to do, and his company went above and beyond to help me achieve my vision.

After that, Coach Z and I took over planning and putting together activity stations,

2010: The first time I met Marcus. This is why I drink milk.

Dad worked with me on the educational stations, and all our Team Tiger experts and volunteers just kept stepping up.

Originally, Marcus just wanted Team Tiger to be the recipient of the proceeds from his gala. But because I wanted to have the camp, Marcus and I agreed on a two-day event, the gala on Friday night and the camp the next morning. It wasn't long before Marcus chimed in again (he's a man of few words, but when he speaks, you listen) and said that the only thing NFL guys like as much as an awesome party is a golf tournament. So now we had a three-day extravaganza!

In the months before the camp, Marcus flew me to Buffalo to see him play, and the structure for the Team Tiger gala/camp/tournament started to develop. During that stay, I went to his house and kicked his butt in *Madden NFL*. (Sorry, Marcus, but the truth must be told!)

As I write this, Dad and I have taken the game plan from that first camp and this book, and we will be doing full camps and mini versions at schools and in NFL cities over the next couple years. I hope to see you at one of my camps.

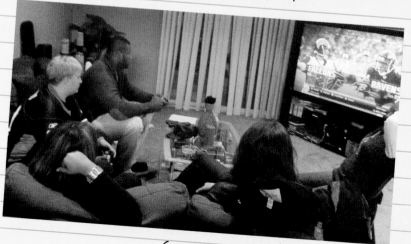

Game on!

Be the Biggest Winner

Probably the question I get asked most often is: What made you finally decide to make this change in your life? To me, though, the real question is: Why didn't I start my journey years ago?

I didn't start sooner because I never felt a connection with any of the so-called experts—doctors on TV and in my community, nutritionists, coaches—who kept telling me how I felt about my weight and what I should do about it. You know that Native American saying about walking a mile in my moccasins? I wish some of these experts could have walked in mine (or jogged twenty yards in my cleats).

I'm not saying they weren't good people. They just didn't know what it was like to be six or eight or ten years old and feel like I did. I always felt that, no matter how many people were around, I was alone and trapped in this giant body. Sometimes I was sad, but I wasn't sure why. I was afraid to get excited about things other kids take for granted—like, I'd worry about taking a piggyback ride from Dad because maybe I would hurt his back. I was afraid to hug or cuddle with Mom, Kaila, or Zack because maybe I'd smother them.

I was even afraid to sit on Santa's lap. I remember being at the mall with my family and some friends around Christmastime—I must have been ten years old. There was Santa, sitting in that big chair with a long line of kids waiting to sit on his lap. I watched as kids my age hopped on without a thought. I wanted to, but I didn't dare. At that point, I weighed two hundred pounds. What if I hurt Santa? What if I rolled off his lap because it wasn't big enough to hold me? (And this is Santa's lap we're talking about!) That was tough. I don't remember crying about it. I just pushed my hurt deep inside. And as usual, I just joked, "Since I'm half Jewish I'd only get to sit on one leg, and that's not big enough."

Watching *The Biggest Loser* wasn't my idea of motivation. (You'll read more about that in the next chapter.) Seriously? This show is supposed to help me? Besides, it's not even for kids.

I needed a role model: a formerly overweight kid talking about how he decided to change his life, someone who could show me that if he could lose weight, I could too. Although I love my parents, family, and friends with all my heart, I needed that kid—guy or girl—who'd walked in my moccasins and felt the same sadness and frustration I did.

Another reason I didn't start my journey much earlier was because, *hello,* I was a kid. If you're an adult, being overweight is usually a direct result of the choices you've made. But mostly, kids get heavy as the result of choices *others* make—choices about what gets put on the breakfast table, their school lunch tray, their dinner plate. Choices about where to go to dinner, what gets put in the refrigerator, the freezer, and the pantry. Adults make those choices, even if we kids fuss and argue about them.

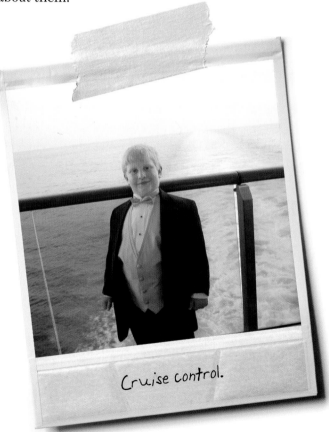

Cruise control.

Am I blaming my parents, or any other adult, for my weight? No way. In fact, I spent most of my life blaming myself. It took a while, but I came to realize that pointing fingers doesn't solve anything or help anyone. For me, change happened when I decided that my future was in my own hands. Even at twelve years old, I could decide to change my life—I didn't have to wait on anyone to decide for me. I had to choose, on my own, to take the next step, make the next right choice, and help everyone around me do the same.

What I really want you to know is that I've been where you are right now. That's why I wrote this book and why I work so hard at Team Tiger. I didn't have a kid to look up to who could tell me how to change. I decided to be that kid.

Find the Tiger in You!

T Totally change your life.

I Inspire those like you and around you.

G Get moving.

E Encourage your family and friends.

R Remember and repeat what you learn in this book.

If you do these things, you'll reap awesome rewards. You'll feel better, physically and mentally. You'll be lighter and faster on your feet, whether you play sports, tag, or ball on the playground; cheerlead; or do dance or gymnastics. You'll be able to wear the clothes you've always wanted to wear. Most of all, you'll have a feeling of pride in yourself.

"Be the Tree" (What?!)

Did you ever have a moment in your life when everything became really clear? When you suddenly understood something that you didn't before? I did—on April 15, 2011, at around six P.M.

It was Friday evening, and Dad, Coach Z, and I were driving to the Ritz-Carlton Hotel in Atlanta, which was hosting a huge party to kick off the camp the next day. It was crazy in that car.

Well, my dad and I were going nuts. Coach Z was totally mellow while Dad was blasting someone on his phone and I was returning emails. This party was a huge deal, and there were tons of last-minute details to take care of. All the way to the Ritz, our phones were blowing up—as soon as we hung up from one call, another would come in.

Earlier that day, we'd planned to get to the hotel early and relax before the party. Well, that didn't work out. The party was starting at six thirty—in thirty minutes!—and we still had all these issues to deal with. Things were getting a little tense in that car.

Then, out of nowhere, Coach Z said something pretty weird: "Be the tree."

That kind of brought us back to earth. My dad gave him a look like, *Are you nuts?* But as soon as Coach Z said it, I totally got it. Then my dad got it too.

As we were flying down the highway, Coach Z explained, this one tree—so small it was almost a bush—caught his eye. It was growing right out of the concrete along the highway. That tree made Coach Z think of me and about the obstacles I faced when I was first starting my journey.

"Who would have thought this tree could make it?" he said. But there it was, pushing up right out of concrete, reaching for the sun. It wasn't an impressive-looking tree. But it was thriving.

Never mind the tree. Who would have thought I would have made it to this night—a pretty big moment in the life of a thirteen-year-old?

So when Coach Z said, "Be the tree," he meant, "No matter what obstacles you face, keep growing."

Do you get it? You're the tree. I'm the tree. In a way, we're all the tree. And no matter what happens in our lives, we can be that tree. We can be strong, overcome whatever life throws our way, stay focused and positive, and succeed, no matter where we start from.

Some trees start out in perfect conditions—lots of sun, great soil—and have an easy time growing and thriving. Some trees don't make it. And some, like the one Coach Z saw, overcome every obstacle—including concrete—to not just survive but also to thrive.

That's my goal: to thrive. To be the best and healthiest me I can be. I hope by the time you finish this book, you see that you too can be the tree.

By the way, that party was over a year ago. I pass that tree a few times a week. It's still there, and it's still growing.

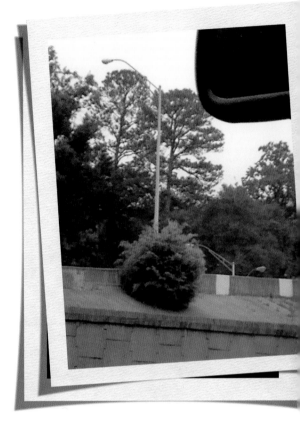

And you think you have it tough!

Your Secret Weapons: Heart and Soul

The first secret weapon is your family. From the moment I decided I would begin this journey (and it was my decision—no one can make it for you!), my family was right there, cheering me on. My family and friends are my soul; they are who I am.

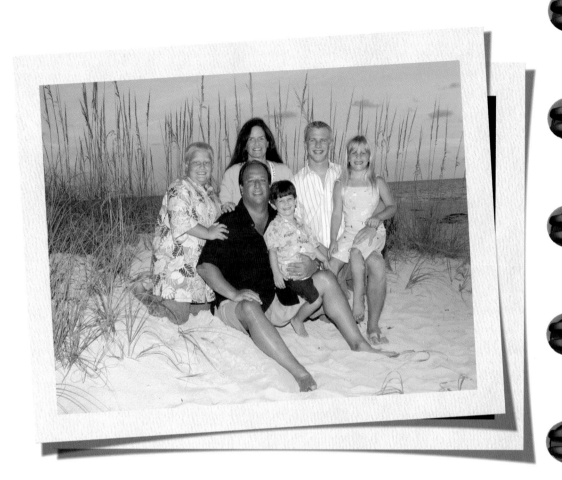

Gang Greene—the original Team Tiger.

Really, you have two families—your own and the Team Tiger family. At Team Tiger we use the term *Ohana*, which is Hawaiian for "family." Coach Z has a house in Hawaii and goes there often (he even has a tattoo of the islands on his leg) and we all love the tropical outdoor life Hawaii brings to mind.

In fact, family is such an important part of success on this journey you're on, I wrote Chapter 3—with a lot of help from Mom, Dad, Kaila, and Zack—just for *your* family. Sit with them as they read it, and talk about what they can do to make your journey easier and more fun. I think your parents, brothers, and sisters—and any other people who are part of your family, whether they are actually related to you by blood or not—will find a lot of ways to support you, as my family and friends have supported me. (In my family, that made Dad an athletic supporter—sorry, that just came out.)

What can your family do? The same simple things my family did to help me. We started eating healthier as a family at home and at restaurants so I didn't feel singled out. My dad stopped making our time together about food. My mom got me running in the mornings, and we entered road races together. My brothers and sisters started asking if everything they were about to eat or drink was Team Tiger–approved, and if it wasn't, they chose a healthier snack or drink. Speaking of drinks—my entire family started drinking water instead of soda. When the journey gets tough, as it sometimes will, it's awesome to have many sets of shoulders to lean on. Your family, and the Team Tiger Ohana, can all "be the tree" for each other.

Your other secret weapon? Coaches call it grit or determination. I call it heart. Heart is your commitment to yourself to always work your hardest, to do your best, to never quit.

One of the best demonstrations of heart I have ever seen was at the dome. There was this little girl (okay, not so little), maybe eight years old, who was first in line at one of our activity stations. When we started the drill, she took off like a shot. But her footwork hadn't quite caught up to her determination, and as she hit one of the obstacles, she did a total face-plant. Before we could react, she hopped up, her face smeared with turf, and finished the drill with a smile. The crowd went nuts. That's heart!

Bottom line: when times get tough, you need to reach deep inside yourself to give 110 percent. The awesome thing about heart is that you've already got it! That's why you're reading this book. And you don't have to take this journey alone. I've taken it too, and I'm still on it—with you.

The Team Tiger Cheer

My whole life, my dad has coached my football team. The team's name is the Green Eagles, but everyone knows us as the Green(e) Machine. Before and after every practice and every game, Dad leads us in a cheer—actually kind of a call-and-respond chant. It goes like this. (Dad calls the lines in the first part; our team shouts out the responses.)

"How many plays do we play?" Every play!

"How many quarters do we play?" Four quarters!

"We play as a . . ." Team!

"We play with . . ." Heart!

To me, this is more than a football chant. It applies to every part of my life, especially to Team Tiger.

Every play is every day I wake up and continue my journey.

Playing four quarters means seeing things through to the end and never giving up, being able to finish what you start and knowing that you fight till you achieve your goals in life. I give my best effort, always. I never give up.

You and me, we're the team.

And everything is possible when you have heart.

So, want to join the team? I'll give you the resources, but only you can add your heart. Once you do . . . welcome to Team Tiger!

The Cheesesteak Story (or: How We Got Our Team Chant)

At age seven, I didn't really play football. I'd play some plays and not others, be tired by halftime, and just kind of deal with the second half. I didn't yet have that drive to win or support my team.

Anyway, we were in a play-off game that year. It was fourth down, and all we needed to do to win was stop the other team. My dad got in the huddle with us and told another kid and me to swap positions. Then he started to pump us up, saying, "We can do this; I believe in you."

In the middle of his motivating, I held up my hand.

"*What?*" he asked, exasperated.

"I can't swap," I said. "The kid on the other team and I have an understanding."

Dad looked at me with a look like, *What?* Then he took the other kid and me by the jerseys and swapped us himself.

Well, we held them—we won. I made the game-winning tackle. After the game, as we were walking off the field, Dad put his arm around me. "What is this 'understanding' you have with this kid on the other team?" he asked.

I explained that if the play wasn't coming our direction, he put two fingers down, which meant we shouldn't try very hard and should save our energy. But if the play was coming our way, he put five fingers down, and we played for real. Dad cracked up.

So at our *next* practice after this game, we were scrimmaging another team. I was doing my usual sitting there—not letting the other team move me but not really playing either. Dad got frustrated and called me off the field.

"What do I need to do to get you to fire off the ball and tackle someone?" he asked.

"Buy me a cheesesteak after practice," I said. I was kind of hungry at that point.

My dad shook his head and barked, "If you get the ball, I'll buy you a Philly Connection franchise." (At the time, Philly Connection was my favorite place to get cheesesteaks. They make, like, twenty different kinds.) ➜

Properly motivated—*cheesesteak! cheesesteak!*—I went up to the line, dug in my feet, and started pumping my butt up and down. When the ball moved, I demolished the center, quarterback, and running back and stood up with the ball in my hands.

My dad's jaw dropped. His assistant coaches' jaws dropped. And from that point on, whenever they needed me to get pumped and make a big play, all my teammates, coaches, and eventually even the crowd would start chanting, "Cheesesteak! Cheesesteak!" My butt would start pumping and, more often than not, I made the play.

That's why Dad and I came up with our Team Tiger cheer. Everyone knows what we and our team stand for: heart. And I learned one of the most important, and most rewarding, lessons of my life because of a cheesesteak.

Granted, they were awesome cheesesteaks.

Cheesesteak!
Cheesesteak!
Cheesesteak!

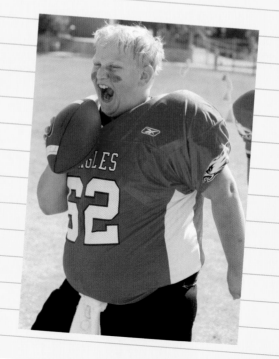

A Peek Inside Your Playbook

At the start of the season, every NFL player gets his team's playbook. A playbook is this spiral-bound notebook, like the kind you use in school, but you don't write in it. This notebook already has the answers. It's a design of how your team will approach each segment of the game. It contains every play and formation the team needs to know to do its best. Everything is clearly drawn so that in the heat of the game, everything is laid out so you can stay focused on what you want to do.

This book is Team Tiger's playbook, and I'm your head coach. This book contains every play I used to lose weight and still use to stay at a healthy weight. Some of my plays involve food. Others involve exercise—what I do to stay active and how I make it fun. And I want you to know this up front: not one of Team Tiger's plays involves dieting or depriving yourself. I didn't get healthy and change my life doing that, and I don't ask you to. Instead, these plays involve making changes that stick, getting healthy, losing the weight for good, and learning to feel great about yourself.

But if a team really wants to succeed, it needs more than brilliant plays in a playbook or even a genius head coach. It needs other coaches—some who really know defense, some who know offense inside and out, and others who coach just linemen or backs.

Well, you're gonna meet five really cool Team Tiger coaches. As far as I'm concerned, these guys are the All-Star team of coaches. All of them came to my camp at the dome to talk about stuff big kids and their parents need to know to start the journey and stay on track.

In part two of this playbook, you'll have four coaches in addition to me. So let's have the lineup!

Dr. Stephen Crabtree (What's Up, Doc?) answers questions that big kids and their parents commonly ask about childhood obesity.

Dr. Linda Craighead (Checkup from the Neck Up) lays out a new play for when you eat. It has to do with the way you *think* about eating.

It's so simple and makes so much sense, you won't believe nobody told you about it before.

Kim Wilson (Eat like a Tiger!) is a registered dietitian who works with professional athletes. She'll coach you on the little changes you can make in what you're eating that will help you lose weight and how to make eating less a no-brainer.

Shane Thompson (Eating Out: It's All About Choices) tells you easy ways to make better choices when you eat at restaurants. Shane probably eats at his own restaurant every day, and I eat there a few times a week, but we've both kept off the weight we lost.

In part three of this book, Coach Z takes over. We've put together a really fun workout routine based on the exercises and drills I do every day. If you've tried to exercise before and given up, this is unlike any workout you've done—because it's actually fun!

But you've still got two secret weapons that will help you start your journey, and play to win!

Yes <u>You</u> Can—Follow Me!

Since that first appearance on *The Dr. Oz Show,* my life has been crazy. Newspaper interviews. TV interviews. Writing this book. It's hard work, and it's not my idea of fun to relive the painful memories I have of being the big kid. But I have to, to get to the fun part: I get to tell big kids that their lives can be different and how they can change. The most important thing to me besides my family and continuing my own journey is to keep spreading the word to big kids and families: yes, we can—follow me!

And people *are* following. Nearly every day, people come up to me at the gym, the Little League park, even the grocery store to tell me that my story has affected them or someone they know. Recently, in the parking lot of a Publix Super Market, a large lady carrying a bag of groceries ran up to Dad and me. "I know I should have parked across the parking lot so I'd walk farther," she said. "But look in my bag—all healthy stuff!" We nodded and high-fived her. (She kind of scared me, but I'm proud of her, whoever she is.)

And a few days ago, one of Kaila's friends, who'd gone to my camp, came to the house. When I last saw her, four months ago, she was pretty heavy. Kaila had told us that her friend had been picked on at school because of her weight (Kaila put a stop to that!), and I could just tell that she felt terrible about herself. Well, I saw her for the first

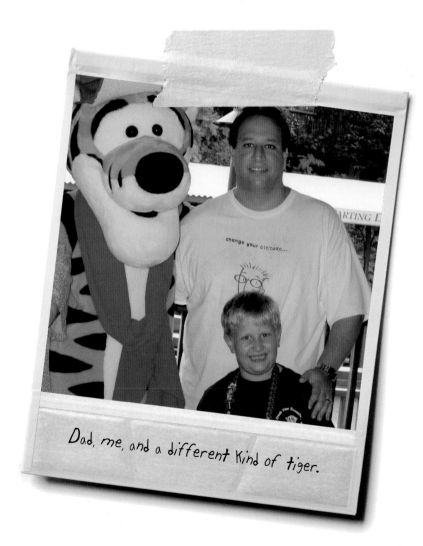

Dad, me, and a different kind of tiger.

time since the dome. Wow! What a difference that four months made! She had lost weight—my guess is about twenty pounds. (I know better than to ask a woman about her weight!) Excitedly, she told Kaila and me about the changes she's made since the camp.

"I used to just hang at the pool all day, soaking and eating," she said. "That's just what we *did*. Now I swim laps. My whole *family* swims laps! I stopped drinking soda—I only drink water now. And instead of buying burgers and fries or ice cream from the snack bar, we bring our own healthy lunch to the pool in a cooler. We walk after dinner too, together. I can't wait to go school shopping—I always hated it before."

I felt so good hearing that. It was like I was back in that tunnel again, watching the kids on the field. I knew that everything I'd been through and all the hard work—getting active every day, changing my eating habits, speaking at schools, giving media interviews about my story, answering the thousands of emails and calls from big kids and their parents from around the country—had paid off.

"You look great," I told her. And she did.

She smiled at me and got kind of teary. I knew what she was feeling right then: pride.

So maybe now you see how Team Tiger works. I lost weight and got healthier and happier, and I'm passing the information on to you and your family so you can do it too. And once *you* do it, you can help others around you get healthier and happier—maybe your mom and dad, one of your friends, or someone you don't even know yet.

By starting to read this book, you've decided either for yourself or for someone you love to begin your journey to a healthier and more active lifestyle. I would like for you to understand how everything contained in this book has changed my life. I've changed from an unhealthy, inactive child into a healthy, active, grateful young man with a nonprofit foundation, Team Tiger, and a mission to help big kids all over the world learn the things I've learned. As you've already seen in the pictures, I've gone through a huge physical change, but so you can understand the complete transformation, let me tell you how my journey began December 8, 2009.

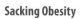

CHAPTER 2

Family, Football, Food... and the Decision to Change

My journey started when I was twelve. We are just finishing dinner—steak, shrimp dip, pierogi, corn on the cob, and garlic broccoli. Dad cooked. We are celebrating: we went down to the courthouse today so I could change my name from Tyler to Tiger. It's been a proud and happy day for me, for all of us, so we're celebrating. With food, of course, as we always do. Actually, dinner is our second celebration meal of the day—after court, we feasted at the best seafood place in Atlanta. When we sat down to dinner, I was still kind of full from lunch, but it's

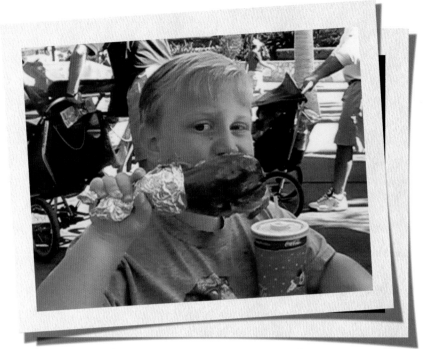

That turkey never stood a chance!

a special day, right? Gang Greene—my dad's nickname for our family as well as our entire extended family—always goes big or goes home, and today is no different.

The Biggest Loser, one of my mom's favorite shows, is airing its finale, so we get up from the table and settle on the couch, bringing our dessert—ice cream sundaes—with us.

I watch for a few minutes—a recap from the previous episode when everyone loses, like, twenty-five pounds in a week. They have so much support—chefs, nutritionists, trainers. Who has a full-time staff to help them lose weight? Who can devote every minute of every day to losing weight?

This show has no basis in reality—my reality, at least.

There's no hope for me.

As I eat my sundae, I start to feel sick to my stomach. I often feel sick from the amount of food I put away, but even though it's my stomach that's reacting, the pain is coming from deep inside.

I look at the people on the television screen and think, *Wow, this could be me. I think this is me.* In my head, I've always known I was big. But now, for the first time, I realize that I am obese.

I get up and head for the stairs. I need to get away from this show. I need to go to my room, stick my face in my pillow, and scream. Might as well take my medicine while I'm up there—six pills a day for diabetes and my thyroid. My knees ache with every step. I lie down and stare at my two bottles of pills on my nightstand. Am I eventually going to need eight bottles, like my dad?

My eyes start to sting. I don't want to be this way. Not anymore.

But how can I lose weight? How can I change my life? How can I save Dad's? Just thinking about it seems overwhelming.

I'm not a contestant on *The Biggest Loser.* I don't have months to do nothing but lose weight. How could that show help kids like me, anyway? The contestants don't have to get up at six A.M., go to school, eat lunch (the school hot lunch, which is anything but healthy), go home, do homework for three hours, go to practice, and get back home at nine or ten P.M. When would I work out? Where would I find the time? And even when I do exercise—during football I run around hitting kids and catching footballs for three hours—I'm starving afterward. I usually beg Dad to stop at our favorite barbecue restaurant so I can grab a quick "snack." How am I going to stop doing that?

Where do I begin?

I'm a tough kid, and I don't cry easily. But tonight, everything is hitting me, and I can't help it. My weight. My dad's health—in a few weeks, he'll go into the hospital for his second heart operation, also because of his weight. And a few days ago, a friend of mine and his mom were in a car wreck. He's in a coma, and I can't imagine how he's going to feel when he wakes up and finds out his mom didn't make it. I feel helpless to do anything about any of it. Another friend of mine just lost his dad to skin cancer. I don't want to lose mine to food.

Life is pretty precious. Weird that I never realized that before. I need to find a way to start taking better care of myself and my family. We all deserve better, and I'm going to make it happen!

The North Carolina Teachers

Minutes before camp started, one of the volunteers running our registration called me onto the field. "Some teachers are here from North Carolina!" she said, kind of breathless. "They said they emailed you but never heard back. But they said there was no way they were gonna miss your camp!"

I laughed. "Okay, they're in," I said. A second later, they started walking down the stadium steps. (You couldn't miss them—they were all wearing blue and yellow T-shirts with cheetahs on them.)

I went to the end of the steps to greet them. "We're so thankful for what you're doing," one said, and the others nodded in agreement. They hadn't been able to convince the 1,200 kids at their school how important it was to eat right and get active now, while they're young. But having seen me telling my story on TV, they knew I could drive the message home. So here they were, ready to learn from me, ready to spread the Team Tiger word.

They were a blast. It was like having a whole group of cheerleaders there taking part in all the stations, absorbing everything, and asking our experts fantastic questions. I later heard that when they got home, they started a mini-camp at their school, based on what they had learned.

These teachers—who gave up their Saturday to travel two hundred miles by bus to learn from me and my team—taught me a valuable lesson. To spread the word about healthy living, it takes passionate, caring people just like them.

And it's not just me. There are kids all over the world who feel like I do right now. And none of us knows what to do.

I hear a knock on my door. My dad pokes his head in. Seeing my dad's big shoulders filling the doorway is usually a comforting sight. But tonight, it doesn't seem to give me any reassurance.

"What's wrong?" he asks.

"Nothing." I don't want to upset him, but I'm not fooling him. He knows me.

"Come on, Tiger. You can tell me anything."

"When are we going to lose weight?" I ask. "You told me it would happen during football. I started this season at two hundred twenty pounds. I'm two hundred fifty now." I know this because our team had to get weighed before the All-Star game, so our weights could be listed in the program. How do you gain thirty pounds playing football?

"Buddy, we'll get to it," my dad says. "We'll get it done."

I know he's trying to comfort me. But there are those words again, the words I've heard so many times from my dad. And I don't believe them anymore.

And so I say, "Dad. That's what you always say."

Dad's head drops, and his eyes are watering. I lift my head off the pillow. I've hurt him. I don't want to hurt him. I love him. It's not his fault I'm two hundred fifty pounds.

It's not his fault.

Suddenly, I'm more furious than I've ever been in my life. I'm not angry at my dad. I'm angry at myself. My dad shouldn't ever have to hang his head because of me. I've been waiting for him, or someone, to make this change for me, but my life and my future aren't only their responsibility. They're mine.

I wipe away my tears and smile. A real smile.

"Stop being a wimp, Dad," I say. "I got this." And somehow, I know I do.

I don't ever want to hear "Don't worry about it" or "You'll grow out of it" again. I'm gonna do it. I'm going to change my life—and save Dad's. I'm going to change the world.

Dial, and Ye Shall Receive (Pizza)

So that was my aha moment—the night when I finally understood that if I was going to change my life, I had to decide to do it, and no one but me could make that decision. But even though I made it in an instant, I was working against twelve years of bad habits and patterns.

Because when I say my family loves to celebrate, I'm not joking. Does serving forty pounds of turkey, plus honey-baked ham, plus steak for Thanksgiving, sound like joking to you? My parents even celebrated my birth with a massive order of Chinese takeout delivered right to the hospital, enough to feed Mom, Dad, Granni, Uncle Larry, Mike, and all the nurses on duty in the maternity ward that night.

Mom tells me I was a normal baby who didn't eat any more than my brothers or sister (although she does recall that my first night out on the town, I sat in my car seat on top of a table at their favorite Mexican restaurant).

I grew into a happy, healthy, strong little guy. And did I mention smart? When I was maybe three years old, I realized that when you told the phone your phone number and address when it asked you for them, a pizza man would soon arrive at the door.

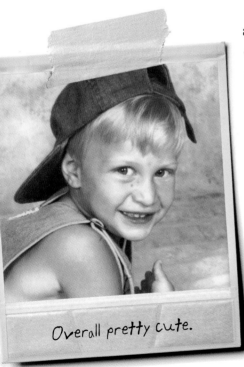

Overall pretty cute.

I had this little table in the kitchen that I used for everything—drawing, eating, playing. One day, sitting at my table drawing, I got bored. So I got up, dragged my table to the counter, climbed up, got the phone, looked at the magnet that had our pizza place's number on it, called the pizza place, and told them my phone number, address, and the kind of pizza I wanted. Then I hung up, went in my parent's room, and asked for a dollar for the pizza guy.

"Sure, buddy, here's a dollar," my dad said, laughing. I took it and went to play with my dog. Five minutes later, I thought it was ridiculous that my pizza hadn't arrived yet, so I grabbed the phone and called the number on the magnet again.

My dad remembers walking into the kitchen and hearing me on the phone asking where my order was. Well, ten minutes later the doorbell rang, and Mom came in, cracking up and telling me that I needed a few more dollars for the pizza guy. That's when my dad realized I hadn't been playing. They both remember being thankful that filet and lobster places don't deliver!

The Story of My Name

I was born Tiger George Greene on September 24, 1997. The next day, I was named Tyler. Then twelve years later, I was named Tiger again. Now that I've totally confused you, let me explain.

When my mom and dad found out the results of the ultrasound—I was a boy—they were watching Tiger Woods play in the Masters Golf Tournament on TV. Okay, Dad was watching. He said, "We'll just name him after whoever wins the Masters." I could have been named Vijay! So from the day Tiger won the Masters, I was called Tiger. My mom says the doctor even shouted, "Here comes Tiger!" in the delivery room.

But here's where "Tyler" comes in. Although my mom and dad had turned in the birth certificate with "Tiger" in the first name box, my mom got cold feet. She thought maybe kids would tease me—little could she know that my name would have no bearing on what kids would tease me about—and that they should give me a "normal" name. So when Dad dropped us off at the house and everyone was waiting there, Mom sent him back to the hospital. With a stroke of a pen, I was legally named Tyler. →

Mom may have won the battle, but Dad won the war. Since the day they brought me home, I have always been called Tiger. The only person I know who has called me Tyler is the registrar at my elementary school (and Mom when she was mad at me)! So on December 8, 2009, my family and I took a celebratory limousine to the Fulton County courthouse to have my name officially changed back to Tiger.

Based on what was going on in the news at this time, I don't know that it was the perfect time for the change. Just weeks before, Tiger Woods got into some trouble. I don't know the whole story, but Dad says that "he ran his car into a tree, and all these women fell out."

But Granni says everything happens for a reason. So when the judge looked at me and asked, "In light of all the publicity the 'other' Tiger is getting, are you sure you want to change your name?" I looked him in the eye and said, "If ever the world needed a Tiger to look up to, it's now."

The immediate perk to the name change is that Mom had nothing official to holler when she got serious! No more "*Tylerrrr!*" Now, she just growls, "Tiiiiiger..."

"He'll Grow Out of It"

While my mom and my brothers and sister never had weight problems, I was always off the growth charts. In kindergarten I was so much bigger than my classmates that my parents went to talk to my teacher about it. This teacher—young and also a high school wrestling coach—put them at ease. "He's not one of those kids who sits around when everyone else is active—he's leading the charge," the teacher told them. Then he uttered those famous words: "He'll grow out of it." I'd hear them a lot over the years.

Yes, I was just a big boy, like my dad. And so I followed in my dad's footsteps. I like to think that my teachers and doctors meant well and that they really did believe I would, at some point, slim down.

But at just eight years old, I weighed 164 pounds. Mom and Dad hired me a trainer. At first, it was cool to have a trainer like the athletes I saw on TV. But when I told the kids in my class, they made fun of me—"You're going to a fat coach," they snickered. After that, the workouts didn't seem so fun or motivating—just hard and boring.

Then I rediscovered football.

Although I'd stopped going to the gym (actually, it closed down, and I didn't join another for a while), my size made me pretty strong for a kid, and that kind of hid the trouble I was in, weight-wise. Finally, I'd found something I was really good at besides eating: football—a sport where after a few seasons I was picked first, not last, where I could hit harder and out-tackle almost anyone on the field. I was also quick footed, able to jump side to side on balance balls effortlessly, something no other kid on my team could do.

What I couldn't do was run a lap around the field. While all the other kids lost weight during football season, working out in full pads in the sweltering summer heat, I kept getting heavier.

Despite my weight, I had gained a lot of confidence and had started to believe I was a pretty good player. But during the 2009 season, something happened during a game that nearly shattered my growing sense of confidence on the field.

Our team was playing our archrivals, the Red Eagles. Their coach had a son on the team. Our favorite play was the Bulldozer Wedge. I played the bulldozer, and our quarterback followed me until someone on the other team stopped us.

We ran this play over and over. The Red Eagles couldn't stop us, and the other coach's son was the recipient of a lot of bulldozing. One time it happened right in front of his bench. As I blocked his son and then

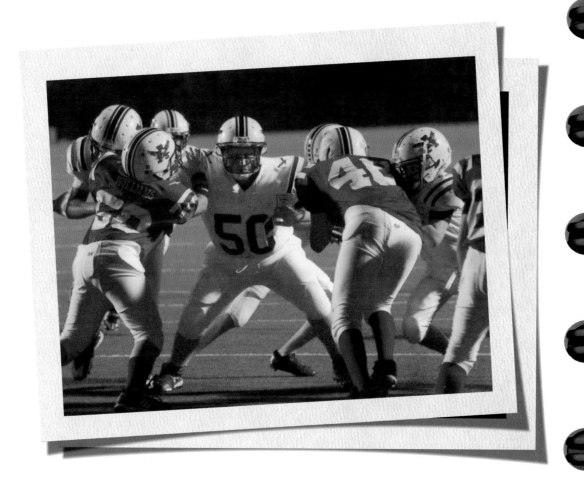

The power of the bulldozer.

fell on top of him, the coach started yelling at me, calling me a glob, and shouting to get off his son. Kids started laughing.

The football field had become my safe haven. But with that one word—"Glob!"—that safe, proud feeling evaporated.

Now I had nowhere to feel good about myself. Anywhere I went—to class, to the mall, out to dinner with friends or family—people stared at me and made comments about my weight. I felt hopeless and defeated. My dad gives a great pep talk, but it just didn't help anymore.

Been There, Tried It— Don't Diet

You might ask, "So why didn't you go on a diet?" I did—lots of them. From the time I started kindergarten. You name the diet, we tried it— Protein Power, Atkins, South Beach, low fat, low sodium, all types of shakes and powders. We'd white-knuckle those tiny portions of rabbit food for a week or two, but then a holiday or celebration would come up, and we'd cheat just a little. Then a little more. Then we would forget to pack my lunch for school, and before long I was back to my old ways.

Not only did dieting feel like punishment, it made me self-conscious. It was like, "Look at the fat kid eating salad." During one of my low-carb diets, a kid passed by my table as I ate my meat-and-cheese roll-ups. "He must have had the rest of the cow for breakfast," he snickered to his friends as they walked by. I wanted to jump up from my seat and knock him out, but I just threw the rest of my lunch away and slouched back to class.

Eventually, sick to death of dieting, my dad and I would sneak off to eat. With practice and games until nine P.M. six nights a week between my team and Zack's, it was easier to pick up fast food or stop in for a late-night dinner at one of our favorite Mexican or barbecue restaurants, where almost everyone knew us. And we loved going out to eat with our team after practices and games. Our favorite wing place actually named one of its private rooms after us: The Greene Room. Once the place knew our games were lasting until ten P.M. or later, it extended its kitchen hours. In we'd come, thirty to forty strong, for our after-game celebrations (we went undefeated that season).

But I was eating more food than I could even digest. Often sick to my stomach, I was spending so much time in the restroom at school that my teachers thought I was trying to cut class. To keep the other kids from making fun of me, I joked that I was "the life of the potty."

When I was in fourth grade, my doctor told my parents that my thyroid had virtually shut down and my blood sugar levels were in the diabetic range. Doctors put me on thyroid medication hoping it would kick up my metabolism. I lost thirteen pounds the first week I was on it, and my dad and I were so happy. But within a week, my system adjusted to the medicine. I went right back to gaining weight and feeling lousy.

In fifth grade I weighed two hundred pounds. In sixth grade, I hit two hundred fifty. I was taking six pills a day for high blood pressure, high blood sugar, and high cholesterol. I stopped breathing for short periods of time in my sleep and woke up gasping for air. My joints ached from the load they had to carry. I was a mess—getting old before my time.

Later on, I found out that I'd had even scarier health problems. The strain of pumping blood through dense fat tissue, my doctor said, had caused my heart to thicken, a condition that can lead to heart failure and heart attacks later in life. My liver was full of fat (now there's a gross visual!), and I had a disease that often causes no symptoms until it destroys the liver.

I was sick and tired of feeling sick and tired. I wanted to be a normal kid who could run and play without pain or exhaustion. But I didn't know how to change—until I had my aha moment.

Yes I Could—and I Did

At that moment I realized that if I was going to have a future, it was up to me to change. But as a kid, I didn't have any role models for how to lose weight. No one under eighteen can go on *The Biggest Loser*. And even if they could, that show wasn't for me.

Yes, my family had once looked to that show for inspiration, but it wasn't exactly inspiring anymore. And it was unhealthy too, the way those people lost weight. Contestants are taken out of their daily lives and put into this artificial environment, where what they eat and how much they exercise is strictly monitored.

Some cast members later confessed to going to extreme lengths to lose weight for the show, using the kind of highly dangerous tactics jockeys and boxers often do to meet weight limits in their sports. After the show aired, one winner blogged about eating not one ounce of solid food for ten days prior to the final weigh-in. Even scarier, he dehydrated himself so severely, by wearing a rubber suit while running on a treadmill and by spending hours in a sauna, that he ended up urinating blood. Only five days after the show ended, he had regained thirty-two pounds just from returning to moderate eating and hydration, and he eventually gained back all the weight he had lost.

I didn't want to be labeled a loser, no matter how the TV show tried to redefine the word as a remarkable achievement. I wanted to be a winner. I didn't want to save just my own life, I wanted to save my dad's and help other families as well. I wanted to be a role model for kids who didn't have weight loss champions to follow, who weren't old enough to join gyms or shop for their own food or control the family menu.

Even at twelve years old, I knew that no magic pill or easy solution would change my lifetime of bad habits. But for the first time, I began to believe that change could happen. I just had to find the way—a way that didn't involve being a loser. In fact, we think all our Team Tiger members are the biggest winners.

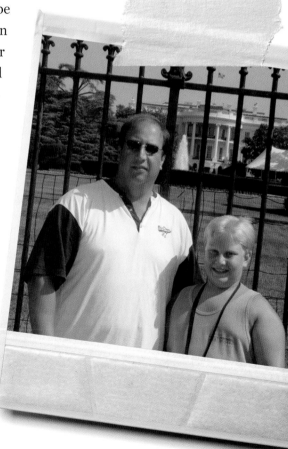

Dad and me in front of the White House. I am a big fan of Michelle Obama's campaign to make kids healthier.

Chalk Talk from Dad: How Parents Can Help

I didn't realize is how my weight and bad health had unmotivated my own son. The night of Tiger's aha moment, I weighed 309 pounds. Sure, I talked a good game about making good choices, but it wasn't until I saw the pain in Tiger's eyes that I knew words weren't enough.

This heavy-duty support did not include dieting with him. I never realized the confusion and shame I caused Tiger with our Diet-of-the-Month Club. Dieting made him feel guilty, ashamed, and weird. Dieting meant that he had to do something his friends didn't.

We discovered that Tiger had a better chance of making healthy food and lifestyle choices if *everyone in the family* ate what he ate and worked out with him. That wasn't hard for Tiger's mom—Marsha had always eaten well and exercised. It was extremely hard for me—I'd had my bad habits longer than Tiger had—but I rose to the challenge. Here's how you can too:

Let your child off the hook.   It's hard to change. Be honest about that. But point out that small changes, like giving up soda between meals, can reap big rewards. Also stress that your children have done nothing wrong—they just have to learn the lifestyle habits that will help them succeed. Tiger always felt guilty, especially if Marsha and I disagreed about his choices. Make sure they know it's not their fault, and be willing to take responsibility so they can start to see the change in you and learn to take responsibility for their own journey.

Pledge your family's support.   How well your family works together as a team can have a huge positive impact on your children's commitment to living healthier. You might gather the family around the table one night after dinner and have each member say what he or she will do to support the team effort. Mom might decide to cook healthier; Dad might say he will stop ordering takeout when it's his turn to fix dinner; all your children might pledge not to bring candy or soda into the house and to eat what the parents serve without complaint. You can do what Tiger did and order brightly colored rubber bracelets and put "Family and Heart" on them in big letters. They serve as a daily reminder of our commitment to each other, and that might work for your family too.

Involve your children in the game plan. Form your plan *with* your children, not *for* them. When Marsha and I discussed how we were going to help Tiger along his journey, he was right there, offering his own suggestions. Put your children in decision-making roles you know they can succeed in. (For example ask, "What shall we have for dinner tonight?" and "Would you rather exercise before school or after?") Tiger loves to pick dinner, so we make sure to narrow the choices so he and the other kids can take their pick and still be healthy. But whether it's chicken or fish, or this restaurant or that, they're making a good choice.

Catch them doing well. Any time you see your children taking a positive action—snacking on a piece of fruit or heading outside to do their workout (see part three)—tell them you're proud of them. And surprise them—blow off that phone call or skip that season finale on TV and make sure they know you would rather be doing something with them.

Don't nag—offer alternatives. Sometimes children don't make the best decisions—perhaps they overeat at a party or skip three workouts in a row. When this happens (and it will), find a positive angle for correction instead of focusing on the negative. When life has gotten in the way and T-bone has skipped a few workouts,

I'll tell him, "Awesome—your body is good and rested, so let's get back at it and do a little more today since we are fresh."

Discuss your challenges openly. If you have ever had weight issues, you know that change isn't easy. Don't pretend it is. If you notice your children struggling with a particular issue, bring it up in a neutral way and then brainstorm ways to solve it. Just make sure they know they are never alone in this journey, either physically or emotionally. You and your children—your entire family—will find a way to succeed.

Be generous with praise. Tell your children often how proud of them you are—and don't forget to toot your own and your family's horn too! Taking pride in your successes lets your kids know that it's okay to feel proud of themselves too.

Be the tree. Remember that from the previous chapter? It works for parents too. Plant those roots firmly, and be strong and steady in your comfort and support.

When your children realize they want to change, it's a cause for celebration. Instead of treating with food, celebrate with praise and gentle support. Never push. Finally, use the lessons of past attempts to build a better future—not just for your children but also for your whole family. I am often aware of the fact that I didn't save Tiger's life—he saved mine.

The First-Quarter Game Plan

I don't remember if I was up all night or slept well after my aha moment, but I found out in the morning that Mom and Dad had stayed up most of the night talking. That morning, December 9, 2009, we sat down at the table together—excited, hopeful, but somehow relieved too. You know that awful feeling you get when you tell a lie? You know that sense of relief when you get busted, because you don't have to live with that awful feeling anymore? It was kind of like that.

We ate breakfast—oatmeal with fresh fruit. I still felt a little hungry, but no big deal. I knew I had started my journey and that it was a marathon, not a sprint. Then we turned to our task: creating our game plan. We called Coach Z, who'd been working with our football team for a year by then, to help us figure out our nutrition and workout plans.

Together, we decided that Coach Z and Mom would tag-team my workouts—he'd work with me several times a week, with Mom working out and running with me when Z couldn't. As for nutrition, we didn't pick a certain diet. We just used common sense. We'd reduce our portions; lay off sugary drinks, desserts, and fast foods; and make healthier choices—all the stuff we already knew (and you may know too). Dad's job was to get through his heart procedure. Afterward, he'd follow the plan with me.

Another big part of my life changed too: school. We found a home-school academy I could go to three days a week for a few hours each day. Without the distractions and demands of full-time school, I could focus on my health but still continue my education. Leaving school didn't bother me at all since I'd still see my friends all the time. (Plus, with homeschooling I got to sleep a little longer!) The owner of the homeschool academy, Mrs. Melinda, understood my mission and became one of Team Tiger's biggest supporters, always helping me keep up with my schoolwork.

After we'd worked out the details, I was pretty pumped—for the first time in a long time. I felt like Dad and I were really going to make it this time. But I wanted to do more. I thought of *The Biggest Loser* again. That show had so many resources for its contestants. But hello, overweight kids need help too! There had to be a way to find support for kids like me.

Then I had a brainstorm. Dad had friends who were NFL superstars. He'd met them over the years through mutual friends and his businesses, and he'd introduced me to some of them. I thought maybe if I wrote to the Atlanta Falcons and to Nike, they'd help me.

I wrote the same letter to both companies. "I have put on 30 pounds this football season alone, and anytime my parents talk to people about help, they don't handle kids," I wrote. "Please help me and I promise I will help lots of other kids learn what I did."

I sent the letters but never got a response. It was clear that I'd have to get started on my own. So I did—and my life has never been the same.

To: Nike
From: Tiger Greene

My name is Tiger, I just turned 12 and live in Alpharetta, GA. I guess I am writing this letter to you because I am scared and don't know what else to do. I have the best parents in the whole world. My dad has coached me and all my friends and classmates for my whole life in baseball and football, and taught us that being part of a team is about so much more than winning or not winning, and because of how close our teams become, I have lots of friends and have met lots of caring athletes. But I am scared because I weigh 250 pounds and can't stop gaining weight. My dad loves me and every time he says we will do something about it something comes up, and we don't stick with it, and I put on more weight. My doctor tells me he loves me too (his son was our QB), but tells me my blood work is getting worse and that we will make an appointment to go over it and then forgets about me or has some emergency and misses my appointment. Everyone says I am the best center and nose tackle but I think it's because of my weight. I have an assistant coach who wanted to do a TV show about me and work with me but my dad says he played in the NFL that doesn't mean he knows how to get me in shape. I see a lot of kids that are big and won't exercise or that don't have friends and get really down on themselves. I am proud of who I am, I just want to be all that I can be and be healthy and safe. I want to show kids that you can be big and proud and that real friends don't care what your weight is, but that you can want to do better and be healthier at the same time. I know it is silly to think Nike would help me, but my dad keeps trying and nothing happens. I have put on 30 pounds this football season alone, and anytime my parents talk to people about help, they don't handle kids. I even asked them if someone like Nike would help sponsor me, could I take the next semester off school and be home-schooled and be able just to work on being healthy so I won't die early like my doctor said could happen, and it's the first time I ever really saw my dad not able to talk. Please help me to "Just Do It" and get healthy and I promise I will help lots of other kids learn what I did. Thanks for listening and I made a disk with some pictures for you.

Nike forever,
Tiger Greene

Tiger G# 99

Believe in Yourself As Much As I Believe in You

When I was three years old, I knew I was bigger than most kids. I didn't know why, and I didn't much care. But other people sure did. Every time I walked into a room or a restaurant or the mall, I got stares, snickers, and sneers. I was a kid, but I always noticed. Maybe you know what I mean—someone turning her head just a little to look over at me or a little kid tugging on his mommy's shirt and pointing. The more years that passed filled with snickers and sneers, the more I started to believe I was guilty of something. I wasn't sure why my weight bothered so many people, but it obviously did.

My confidence disappeared. I became shy around strangers, and even though I was lucky to have some good friends, I never wanted to be far from home. My mom has a horse term she used for me: *herd bound*, which means I always wanted to be with my family. I never slept over at a friend's house—ever. I was afraid that I might not fit in their bed or shower or I wouldn't get enough to eat. So they slept at my house.

Once I began getting pretty good at football—which took time because my size had always been such a negative factor—I started to realize, with the help of some of

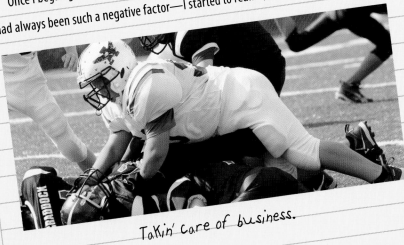

Takin' care of business.

my close friends, that it was okay to find positive traits about myself. Most important: my sense of humor and love of life. Next: my ability to shed my shyness and be a leader. These two positives started to shape the rest of my turnaround.

I became proud of who I was. Although I realized I had to make changes, I didn't care about blame, only about positive change. I started to allow myself to work toward my potential.

Every single one of the kids I've met on my journey has something special and unique about them—a great sense of humor, a brilliant mind, or simply being the best sibling or son or daughter they could be. I'll bet you have that something special too—you just have to find your strengths and take pride in them so you can build on them. Maybe most of all, you have to believe in yourself—know that your journey is worth starting. And if you can't do that this very second, no worries. I'll believe in you until you can believe in yourself.

Now It's Your Turn

The other day, I met with a reporter who interviewed me about my journey and Team Tiger. Afterward, Kaila, who'd hung out with me during the interview, floored me with a great question—better, actually, than any the reporter had asked.

She asked me, "Tiger, if you could turn back time so that you'd never been heavy, would you?"

The answer seems like a no-brainer, right? But then I remembered the last eighteen months. Thought about the thousands of emails, from all over the world, I've received, the thousands of kids and parents I've met, the stories they've told me.

"I wouldn't change a thing," I said. And it's true. This journey, and the tough times I got through, have made me who I am, and I'm proud of who I am. I have gone from a follower to a leader, from snickers and sneers to pats on the back and high fives, from living to eat to eating to fuel my passion for life, and from being unsure and shy to confident and life-loving. That's why I'm telling my story. Maybe if you think about how it's like yours—how I'm like you—you will find it easier to believe in yourself and in your ability to change your life.

One thing I've learned is that once you start this journey, it never really ends. I'm still on mine, still learning about health, my body, and myself. But the great thing is, you never have to take this venture alone—so many people are on it. Although this journey we're on may take us to different places, we can still take some of the same paths.

Because when I say, "Yes we can—follow me," I mean it. I have felt and struggled with most of what you feel and struggle with— the sadness and the anger, the hurt and the loneliness. Now I'm here to help you through it. If you have a question or need to vent, I'm only an email away. We have Team Tiger members who are as young as four and as old as . . . well, let's just say really old with lots of grandkids.

I'm no skinny goalpost, and odds are I never will be. But I am healthy, energetic, and happy, and you can be too. Every bit of the information I share

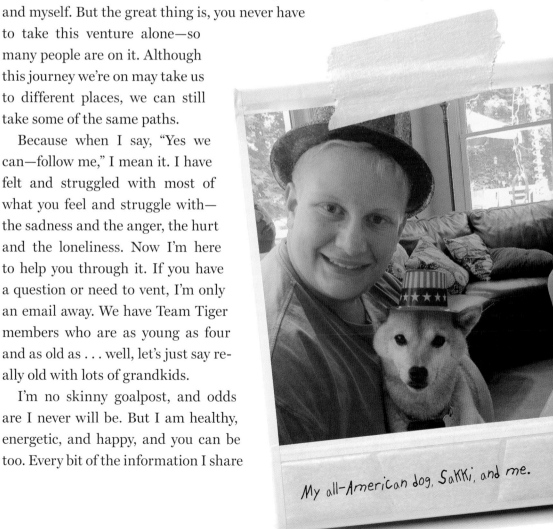

My all-American dog, Sakki, and me.

in this book, about making better food choices and getting more active, comes straight from my own life. It can help you lose weight, improve your health, and feel more positive, right from the very first tough-to-get-started moments.

You can win this battle, just like I have. And if you get snickers and sneers like I did, I promise you that eventually they'll become pats on the back. You don't need to be lectured or have life explained to you—you have probably experienced more heartache than most average adults.

Just take a deep breath and give
yourself a chance. And if you feel hopeful and
maybe even a little excited, awesome!
You're about to start something big, and
you're going to bring everyone
you love along for the ride!

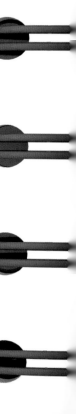

PART 2

Follow Me Into ...Eating Healthy

Am I gonna ask you to go on a diet? Nope. Tell you that you can't eat your favorite foods ever again? Get real! What I am gonna do, with the help of some pretty smart experts, is teach you new ways to think about food and eating. Chill out, though. We'll do this to-gether, and remember: if I can do it, so can you.

I live in a city full of doughnut shops, burger joints, and pizza places—there's food everywhere you go. I also grew up eating pretty much whatever I wanted, whenever I wanted it. It took years for me to build up my bad habits. The two biggest problems for me were that I ate too much food, and the foods I chose weren't the healthiest. So what I learned to do, with the help of my family and the experts I mentioned, is to eat less and make healthier choices.

As I made these changes, my attitudes toward food changed. It was amazing how much of my life I got back when I stopped planning my days around my meals. Instead, food just became the fuel for my adventures. The greasy, fatty foods I once craved don't really appeal to me now. My taste buds seem to have changed, or maybe just my mind-set has. A once-favorite chocolate dessert now tastes too sweet; the flavored popcorn I used to love seems too cheesy. Managing my portions isn't hard anymore—I just think about how much work I've done and I don't want to undo it. I can have one piece of pizza without eating the whole pie, as I used to do. I even chose to have a healthy birthday celebration—instead of cake and ice cream for my thirteenth birthday, I had chocolate-dipped strawberries. If I really want a treat, I let myself have a bite and then ask myself: worth it or not worth it? Eat to live, don't live to eat—that's the way I roll now.

You probably already know how to eat healthy. But knowing how to do it doesn't mean it's easy to do it, especially when you're not used to doing it. But think of it this way: learning to make healthy choices is just like learning any other new skill—riding a bicycle, playing the guitar, or mastering a video game. Those skills take practice, and making better food choices takes practice too.

When I started my journey, I didn't know anything about eating healthy (or at least I didn't think about what I probably knew). But I was determined to lose weight, save my life and my dad's, and live a longer, happier, healthier life. Am I the skinniest kid on the block? Nope. But I'm healthier and happier, and I can't imagine any other way to live—or eat.

To lose weight, you have to learn these skills. This is the part of the book that helps you learn them. And because I know it's a drag to worry about nutrition all the time, I've figured out some shortcuts. You'll learn them in this section.

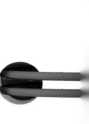

CHAPTER 3

What's Up, Doc?

Have I shared how much I used to hate needles? Because of the medical issues caused by my weight, I had to get a lot of blood work done. The doctors needed to check my blood sugar and my thyroid levels. The problem was that I wouldn't let them take my blood for six years, until I was eleven.

It's not that they didn't try. The only people who hated needles more than I did were the doctors and nurses who tried taking what was rightfully mine: my blood. To stop them, I barricaded the door. I ran out of the examining room and into the hallway in my underwear. (Now you understand why *they* hated needles too!) I chased the doctor out of the room and slammed the door on his assistant's foot. No, I did not like needles. (I still don't, but now I know they're part of this journey at times.)

Considering my behavior, it's no wonder doctors stopped asking for my blood and began to give my parents and me the now-famous medical diagnosis: "Don't worry about his weight. He'll grow out

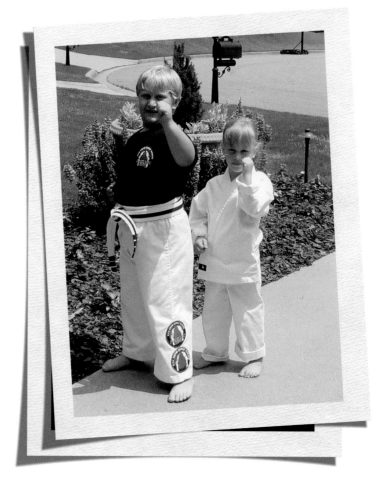

Kaila and me in fighting stance. I'm still fighting—for kids' health!

of it." Or, even better, "No worries. He's just built like his dad. He's gonna be a big boy."

You'd think with all the childhood obesity drama in the news, doctors would know better than to say stuff like this. Well, check this out. Last year, my dad took Kaila for her ten-year-old physical. The doctor had seen me on TV. He asked all about Team Tiger. And then, during Kaila's checkup, the doctor checked her height and weight. Kaila was in the 90th percentile, he said. That meant she was bigger and taller than 90 percent of girls her age, but she's always been that way.

And then, without skipping a beat, the doctor said, "But don't worry—she'll grow out of it." I swear, I can't make this stuff up. I asked Dad what he said to the doctor. "I told him that you were writing a book and it was called *He'll Grow Out of It.*"

Okay, so not all doctors can get real. But you can. Isn't that why you picked up this book? You know you need to make a change. So ask your parents to find you a doctor who cares enough to be honest with you and to help you on your journey. They are out there. In fact, I have one.

His name is Dr. Crabtree, and I met him at about the same time I began my journey. In fact, he spoke at my first camp at the Georgia

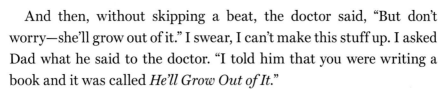

Meet the Team Tiger Expert!

Stephen Crabtree, DO, FACEP

I first met Tiger when my son Braden was playing AYFA football. They started off as rivals, but through a series of events and with Tiger's dad's help, they ended up on the same team and have been friends ever since.

With the help and support of his family and his community, Tiger has accomplished what millions of overweight kids dream of doing—but it doesn't have to be just a dream. Tiger's message is simple: eat right, exercise, expand your mind, and be dedicated to something. Have a purpose. Seek the help you need—it's out there. Let this book guide you to a better place. A healthier place. A happier place. And a more fulfilling place.

> Dr. Stephen Crabtree graduated from the Oklahoma State University College of Osteopathic Medicine in 1993. Upon graduation, he completed a four-year residency in emergency medicine at the University of Oklahoma Health Sciences Center and went into clinical practice.
>
> In 2005, he became associate professor at the Medical College of Georgia (now Georgia Health Sciences University). Currently a partner in clinical practice in Atlanta, Dr. Crabtree also provides medical support and guidance to local athletic teams.

Dome. To know that I had a friend and a doctor a phone call away got me through some tough situations.

This chapter includes the most common questions that kids and their parents who've come to my camp have asked. Although I wrote the answers, they've been reviewed by Dr. Crabtree, so you get Dr. Crabtree's expertise just like I did. Of course, you may also want to run this information by your own doctor.

Your doctor might not become a great friend like Dr. Crabtree has to me (especially if you inflict bodily harm on him or his assistants when they're in pursuit of your blood), but he can be part of the solution. Don't be afraid to ask questions. More important, don't be afraid of the answers. (You may not like those answers, but—unlike pizza rolls—they are the start of your new, healthy way of life.) And by the way, should you ever need blood work, ask for a little freeze spray. You'll never even feel the needle.

Was I just born to be big?

I have learned that heredity plays a part in obesity. If one or both of your parents are overweight, you may be more likely to be overweight too, especially if there are always chips, cookies, soda, and other high-fat, high-sugar foods at home.

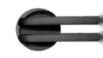

But my journey has taught me three things: 1) I wasn't "born" to get as heavy as I did, 2) getting that heavy doesn't happen overnight, and 3) it can be stopped—if you know what the signs are and what to do about them. And you're learning these in this book.

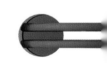

I didn't come into this world any larger than the average baby. I weighed 7.5 pounds and was twenty-one inches long. But I was born into a family that celebrated everything with food—and boy, did we celebrate!

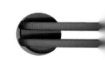

There are red flags that increase anyone's—even kids'—likelihood of becoming heavy. Look at the list below. Do you see any of these flags in your own life?

What you eat. If most of your diet is made up of foods that are high in sugar and fat, you are more likely to gain weight. These foods include fast food, cookies, candy and other sweets, and sugar-sweetened drinks—even sports drinks!

Because you're a kid, you probably don't do the cooking and shopping, so when you consider how you eat, you also have to consider how your parents eat. Do you come from a family of big eaters like I do? Does your family eat on happy occasions, sad occasions, or no occasion—just because that's the way it is in your house? I am not asking these questions to make you or your parents feel guilty. I am asking them so you can become more aware of the choices you make, just like I did.

How much you move. Whether you live in a pineapple under the sea, spend too many hours in front of Nickelodeon, or spend too much time working on the double reverse on *Madden*, you ain't burning enough calories, baby! Odds are, if you are rackin' up the points, you are packin' on the pounds.

Even if you're pretty active, if you eat too many high-fat or high-sugar foods, you can get heavy. Believe me, I know. I put on thirty pounds in one football season—that's four months! And we practiced two hours a day, five days a week, in hundred-plus degree heat. Other kids lost eight to fifteen pounds, and I put on weight!

Even though I was playing a lot of sports, I ate more food than my body needed for energy. When I started to make healthier choices and watch my portion sizes, I lost weight. It's very important that you keep this rule in your mind at all times—we've got to burn at least as many calories as we take in.

Your family tree. Like I said, if one or both of your parents are heavy, you're more likely to follow in their footsteps. That doesn't mean you're doomed. I say it just so you can be aware of it. And you and your family can break the cycle, if you're determined enough. If you have any doubt about that, look at my dad and me— between the two of us, we've lost more than a hundred pounds.

 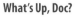

Don't wait for your parents or count on them to start you on your journey. You are in charge of your own health and future, and you have to live with the consequences. So be willing to be the match in your family that lights this candle so that you can all see clearly.

Your emotions. I can't say that I used to eat to cope with stress or because I was bored, sad, or lonely. But I've learned that many kids do, and I've met a lot of them—not just at my camps but also in my neighborhood and schools and Little League parks. And doctors now know that how you feel about yourself and what's going on in your life can definitely influence how much you eat and the food choices you make. Fortunately, there are ways to cope with those issues. In Chapter 4, you'll learn an easy way to stop automatically reaching for food when you're not hungry. I know this sounds like stuff you've heard most your life, but I'm gonna tell you what worked for me—and I'm going to do it in a way that only kids like us who've been there can relate to.

People tell me that I will grow out of being overweight. Can't I just wait until then?

That's what doctors told me—over and over again. For a long time, my family and I all believed the doctors who said that, although my weight was off the charts, I would grow out of it—or into it. Yeah, right.

Looking back, I think maybe doctors don't want to use the word *obese* when talking about a child because they don't want to offend the parents and lose a patient. Fortunately, one doctor did have the courage to say that my dad and I were obese. I still remember my dad's doctor, Dr. Knopf, telling him that he and I were digging our graves with our teeth. That comment sticks with me to this day. I don't think I'll ever forget it.

In his study of childhood obesity, Dr. Crabtree has learned that kids who are chubby sometimes do slim down as they hit puberty simply

Chalk Talk with My Mom: What Parents Can Do

I remember my first inquiry at the pediatrician's office about Tiger, then three years old, who was quickly and obviously becoming heavier and bigger around the middle.

"He's getting pretty big, Doc," I said. "Should I be worried? Should I do something different?"

The doctor answered my question with a question: "How is his dad? Big, you say? Oh, he's just built like his daddy. It's genetics."

Really? Seriously? If I had known then what I know now, I would have pushed my question further or sought a second opinion. Genetics is *not* the cause of childhood obesity. It certainly can be a contributing factor, but the family's lifestyle, habits, food choices, and portion sizes are major players in the weight game.

If you're concerned about your child's weight, don't settle for a simple, unhelpful answer from your pediatrician. He or she should at least be able to tell you the average weight for your child's age or the proper caloric intake based on height and weight. You might also talk to another parent who has a heavy child. Find another pediatrician. There are doctors out there who focus specifically on overweight kids, who know how to answer your questions and how to help your child or children. They can refer you to other specialists, for example a nutritionist or nutritional psychologist. Eventually, we found specialists who were recommended to us. They knew what Tiger needed and didn't treat him as a little adult, but as a child.

Never stop learning or asking questions. If there's one thing I have learned over the years, it's that while parents aren't perfect, doctors aren't either. By definition, they are *practicing* medicine, so it's our job as parents to keep asking the questions and to not be afraid of the answers.

because they're growing so fast. But if they don't change the lifestyle habits that made them heavy kids—if they don't eat healthier foods, watch their portion sizes, and get active—they will gain the weight back as they get older.

Why go through all that? Start living healthier today. If you learn to eat healthy and make exercise a habit, you'll lose the weight now—and you'll be able to keep it off for the rest of your life.

Could I be heavy because of a health problem? Should I get a checkup before I go on your program?

There are some health issues that can cause childhood obesity—they have to do with your family tree (that is, genetics) or hormonal problems. But not many kids have these conditions. Most of the time, we get heavy because we take in more calories than we burn. Fortunately, there's a cure for that: eat healthier and move more. If you take a look at my before and after photos, you can tell I figured it out!

Doctors typically advise adults to get a checkup before they start a weight-loss program just to make sure they don't have any health or medical issues that might crop up as they eat healthier and increase their physical activity. It's not a bad idea to ask your mom or dad to call your doctor and find out if they should check you out before you start my program. Follow their advice. If you do go, ask your doctor these questions, or any other questions you may have about your weight and health, and see what he or she says. The more you know about weight gain, the better equipped you are to change it!

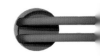

Why do I feel tired all the time?

I asked Dr. Crabtree this question myself, and he said that there are a couple reasons big kids feel tired. First, they might be eating too much unhealthy food made with white flour and white sugar. These types of

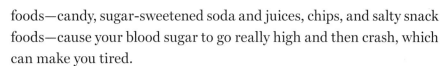

foods—candy, sugar-sweetened soda and juices, chips, and salty snack foods—cause your blood sugar to go really high and then crash, which can make you tired.

Another reason you're probably tired is because you're not getting enough activity. As weird as it sounds, the more active you are, the more energy you have, but the less you move, the more tired you feel. And although only a doctor can tell you for sure, a thyroid problem or high blood sugar might be the cause of your fatigue.

When I was at my heavier weights (as you might remember, my top weight was two hundred fifty pounds at five feet tall), I was tired all the time too. I was carrying extra weight, and I didn't move much because I always felt lousy and my joints were killing me. The fact that I didn't eat breakfast didn't help. Think of your body as a car. Your body burns fuel every second of the day to keep itself running and, while you sleep, to make repairs. After eight hours of sleep and no food, you need to refuel. Breakfast is that fuel.

I didn't know that then, though. With no fuel in my body, I would be exhausted when I got to school and I often dozed off during my morning classes. By lunchtime, I was starving! After a huge lunch and an equally big dinner, I didn't have the energy to do my homework and I was often so stuffed and miserable, I just wanted to sleep.

Regardless of the cause, the solution is to change your lifestyle. It's pretty simple: eat smaller meals, more often, and be active every day. You don't have to diet or run marathons. Take it from me—small steps, like those you'll learn in the coming chapters, lead to big results. Pretty soon, your family is going to look forward to your getting them outside to play. Or maybe you'll run laps in your dad's office like I do if I don't get my exercise in for the day.

Why do my joints always hurt and I always feel sick?

Oh, man, I remember how much my joints hurt. It's because being heavy puts stress on your knees, ankles, and hips—joints that nature didn't design all that well in the first place. (Dr. Crabtree says that even though we walk on two legs, not on all fours, we aren't actually designed that well for walking upright.) The increased weight causes your joints to swell, much like how the joints of older people who have arthritis swell. This swelling is what hurts.

Feeling sick all the time is caused by a not-so-healthy diet. Maybe you're not getting enough fruits and vegetables, and it's hard to go to the bathroom. That can make you feel bloated and sick to your stomach. It's possible that your gallbladder could be acting up too—gallbladder disease used to be something that only older people suffered from, but more and more overweight kids are experiencing it. Of course, only a doctor can tell you that—which is maybe a good reason to get checked out before you start your journey.

What is type 2 diabetes, and what is my risk?

Dr. Crabtree tells me that type 2 diabetes and being heavy go together like peanut butter and jelly. In the past, it was mostly overweight adults who got it. Today, more kids are diagnosed with it, probably because more kids are overweight. I was really close to having it myself. I had what's called metabolic syndrome, which is one step away from full-blown type 2 diabetes.

When you have type 2 diabetes, your body has a problem using its main source of energy—a kind of sugar called glucose. Your body makes glucose from the food you eat. When people eat, glucose moves into their bloodstream. Then a hormone called insulin, made by an organ called the pancreas (which looks kind of like a tadpole), helps push that glucose into their cells so their bodies get the energy they need.

But if you have type 2 diabetes, insulin can't do its job very well. Without insulin to push the glucose into your cells, it just hangs out in your bloodstream, where it builds up. Your pancreas cranks out even more insulin to try to get that glucose into your cells, but eventually it just can't. It's worked too hard for too long making all that extra insulin. So your blood sugar levels rise too high, which makes you sick.

The tendency to get type 2 diabetes is probably passed down through families, Dr. Crabtree says. So if your mom or dad has it, you're more likely to get it. Kids who are African American, Hispanic/Latino, or Native American or who come from an Asian/Pacific Island background are also more likely to get it.

But don't freak. Even if you're big now, you can decrease your risk of getting type 2 diabetes just by getting to a healthy weight and being active. And you can do that if you follow me!

My friend keeps telling me I should stop eating so I'll lose weight. She says that because I'm so big, not eating for a couple days or weeks is okay. She says she does it once in a while to keep her weight down, and she seems okay. Should I take her advice?

Are you kidding me? You should run from that advice. (That's one way to get cardio!) It's true that being heavy can hurt your health. But even if you're a big kid and need to lose weight to get healthy, not eating for days at a time, or deciding to eat only salads or something stupid like that, could hurt your health even more.

When people diet, they're trying to eat fewer calories than their bodies use. By doing this, they may lose weight. But kids usually do not need to diet in this way (or in any way). I don't do diets. I do lifestyle change. So you definitely should not starve yourself or go on those crazy diets you find on the Internet. Your body is still growing, and you need enough food—healthy food—to grow properly. Even if you're heavy, you can probably lose weight by eating only when you're hungry—you'll find out all about that in the next chapter—and by being more active, which you'll also learn all about.

Plus, as weird as it sounds, you have to eat to lose weight. That's because when you eat only one meal a day, or nothing at all, your body actually thinks it's starving to death so it holds on to its energy stores because it doesn't know when to expect food again. That means that even though you're eating almost no calories at all, you won't burn them off and you'll gain weight! Plus, you'll probably get really tired, have terrible headaches, and be so incredibly grouchy that even your dog will avoid you.

Diets that don't include a variety of nutritious foods or that have too few calories can be dangerous for anyone, but in my opinion, given what I have learned about health during my journey, they're especially dangerous for kids. Let me say this: if you're eating nothing but cabbage soup, you're on a dangerous diet. If you don't eat any fat or any carbs, you're on a dangerous diet. I could never stick to diets like

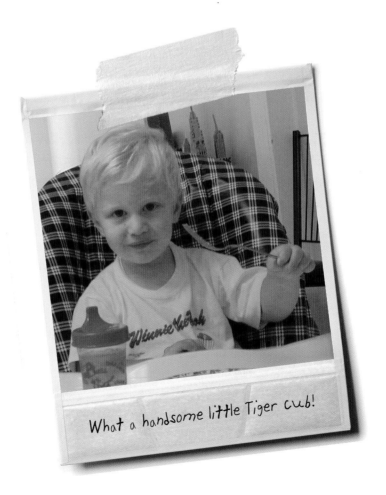

What a handsome little Tiger cub!

this because even though I don't eat as much as I used to, I still love food. Food is not your enemy. You just have to learn how to eat in a healthy way.

What about those pills advertised on TV to burn fat? Would those work for me? (Also, are they safe?)

How great would it be if you really could take a pill, eat anything you want, and still lose weight? It would be totally awesome. But no matter what the TV commercials or the magazine ads say, there is no pill that you can buy over the Internet, or in the drugstore, that can do that. When it comes to losing weight, the only thing that really works is eating less and moving more. Those pills don't work. The only weight you'll lose is in your wallet.

While those so-called fat-burning pills don't work, there's one thing they can do: make you sick. Given their effects, I can't believe that they are safe. They can make your heart pound like a jackhammer and can also make you feel nervous, dizzy, and weird. Please don't let anyone tell you that these pills work. If they did, wouldn't every heavy person on the planet be thin by now?

The idea of doctor-prescribed diet pills and surgery may be tempting as a quick fix. But Team Tiger is about changing how you live and how you think so hopefully you never have to even consider those options. And let's be honest—wanting the easy or quick way out is the same mentality that got many of us to this point.

I'm pretty big. How can I lose weight if I'm too heavy to exercise?

Dr. Crabtree says that the answer to this question is that being heavy makes getting active difficult but not impossible. That's certainly true—I did it—but there's much more to say.

To me, this question hits home with so many of us, especially me. This was what I always told myself—and my coaches and teachers—so I wouldn't have to exercise. Don't get me wrong—I wasn't trying to make excuses; I truly believed I was too big to exercise, and I was concerned about it. But now I see it was my biggest excuse of all.

Earlier, you read about December 8, 2009—the date of my aha moment—and how badly my knees and joints hurt just walking up the stairs to my room. Well, the morning of December 9, I got up at six A.M. and joined my mom in the kitchen. After a healthy breakfast, we

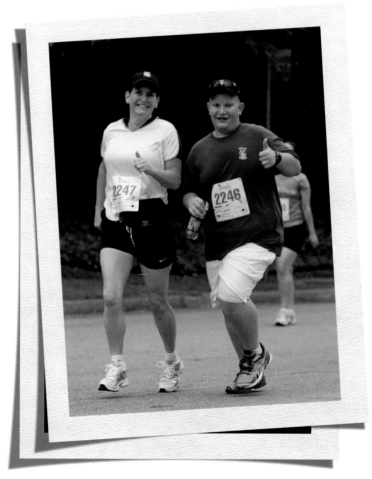

My mom and me on my first 5K.
Who would have thought?

headed out for our first run together—and boy, do I use the word *run* loosely.

We jogged out of our short driveway and up the street at a good clip. By the time we got to the first cross street forty yards from my house, I had to stop jogging and walk. But I didn't quit. I just kept alternating walking and jogging. By the time we got home, about forty-five minutes later, I'd covered a little over two miles. I was sore but proud. We walked/jogged again a few days later. And a few days after that.

Eventually, I started walking/jogging 5K races (which are 3.1 miles long). And in July 2010, I crossed the finish line of the Peachtree Road Race with my mom. I didn't jog the whole way—I was also playing in hydrants and dumping cups of water on Mom when she wasn't looking—but I finished the race. Kaila and Zack came running up to the finish line and told me Dad was in tears, but they didn't need to tell me. I saw his pride, and those tears, when I walked up to him at the end of the race and he kissed my head and hugged me.

So don't use your weight as an excuse—yes, I said excuse. No matter how big you are, take the first step, no matter how small.

Big Kids, Big Health Problems

There are lots of reasons kids want to lose weight, but I would say that kids are more worried about the ABCs of being a big kid: Alone and Afraid, Burgers and Bullies, and Clothes and Comments. It was Dr. Crabtree (along with some other experts) who explained to me how being heavy can impact kids' health—not when they're forty but right now.

Besides insulin resistance and diabetes, here are a few of the health problems that can affect overweight kids and teens:

- Arthritis. Extra pounds can cause wear and tear on your joints and can lead to this painful joint condition pretty early in life.

- Asthma. Obesity is associated with breathing problems that can make it harder to keep up with your friends, play sports, or even just walk to your classes.

- Fatty liver. It's so gross, but basically, fat accumulates in the liver and can cause the liver to swell. It can also scar the liver and lead to permanent damage.

- Gallstones. These happen when bile, a fluid secreted by your gallbladder, forms into hard little pellets in the gallbladder. I've never had gallstones, but I've heard that they're extremely painful. You might even need surgery to have them taken out.

- High blood pressure. When you have high blood pressure, as some big kids do, your heart has to pump harder and your arteries must carry blood under greater pressure. If the problem isn't fixed, your heart and arteries may no longer work as well as they should.

- High cholesterol. Heavy teens may have abnormal blood lipid levels, including high cholesterol, low HDL ("good") cholesterol, and high triglyceride levels. These increase the risk of heart attack and stroke as you get older.

- Sleep apnea. This is when you stop breathing for seconds—or even minutes—when you sleep, and it's a serious problem for many overweight kids and adults. If you have it, you might feel tired all the time, like I did. It can also affect your ability to concentrate and learn, and may eventually lead to heart problems.

That's one long list. But don't freak out—I'm not trying to scare you. As you get healthier and more active, many of the health issues you may be dealing with now will improve or outright reverse themselves. You have your whole life ahead of you, and time is on your side. If you start your journey now, you'll be able to say (as I always do), "I got this," in a year or less.

Chalk Talk from My Parents: Kids Need *You!* (Whether You're a Parent, Stepparent, Grandparent, or Guardian)

We have four kids ranging in age from eight to twenty-five, and one thing that never changes for us, regardless of our kids' ages or sizes, is that we never stop loving or protecting them. So keep the following simple points in mind, whether you're in the pediatrician's office or talking to your children on the phone. (Whether you're a mom or dad, grandparent or guardian, you can still give your children the support they need— individually and by enlisting the help and support of family or friends.)

It's your responsibility to get the best care for your big kids—don't let them down!

M Make a list of questions and concerns.

O Overemphasize your children's medical and emotional symptoms so they are not taken lightly.

M Minimize the drama and scare tactics some doctors use and communicate on a level your children can handle at that point in their journey.

D Don't let your pediatrician get away with a cookie-cutter diagnosis or generic comments (like "He'll grow out of it").

A Allow for a balance of reality and compassion, and always make sure your children know you are taking this journey together.

D Distinguish between treating your children because of a health condition (such as high blood sugar or an underactive thyroid) and letting doctors medicate your children to better health because it's easier than making lasting lifestyle changes.

Why do I need to know all this health stuff anyway?

Because knowing it can help you change your life.

It's hard to feel good when your body has too much weight to carry. Being overweight can make you feel tired all the time and cause aches or pains. It's hard on your emotions too. When you're really heavy, you don't feel all that great about yourself, and you might feel embarrassed, sad, or angry all the time. Or you may even always act silly to divert attention to what you are doing rather than how you look. So there are a lot of reasons to learn how you can lose weight in a safe, healthy way.

But you don't have to do it alone. Getting help is important. That's what you're doing by reading this book, so you're already on your way! Right here, right now, you can take control of your health and let your parents and doctors know that you want to change. And you need to know all this health stuff so that you, with the help of your parents and your doctor, can create a plan for success. You have to know what you need to improve on and then get to it. If I can do it, so can you. If you follow me, don't be surprised at how many other lives you change along the way!

How can I change? How can I get my parents involved and active with me?

You're the only person who can make the decision to change. But at the same time, you need help to get started, and that's what parents are for. I had to tell my dad that I didn't need a friend, I needed a dad (and a mom too) to help me make the right choices and to take temptation out of the house. I needed to tell them that it was okay to tell me no. As in, no, you can't order three appetizers. No, one soda is enough. Hey, I may be talking to friends, but I heard your order and no, the nachos grande are just too grande. We needed a Nike shirt that said, "Just *Don't* Do It!"

It was hard for my parents to say no, but they did it—for me—and it was the single greatest act of love they could have shown me. They helped me become a kid again—a kid who once again has a healthy, active life in front of him.

We can all do it together. That is family at its finest, and the whole gang needs to get into the act. Start going shopping with your mom or dad, and pick out healthy foods and snacks together. Heck, you and your brothers and sisters (if you have them) might even start helping to make dinner every night. Try healthy foods you've never tried, like sushi. Try to make a decent-tasting side dish or dessert out of a vegetable or fruit you've never tried. Get your family out of the house after dinner and go for a family walk. While you're watching TV at night, hold contests (who can do the most crunches during one commercial?). The more involved your family is, the more fun this whole journey becomes. All of a sudden, getting healthy isn't a chore. It's something you do together.

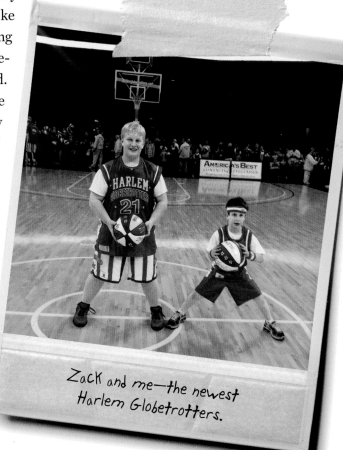

Zack and me—the newest Harlem Globetrotters.

I've been through a lot of doctors and pediatricians throughout the years. And every time I went to one of them, it was pretty much the same old story: "We've got to get you on a diet," "You need more exercise," and "You'll grow out of it." And the thing is, I think they really meant well. But in the ten or fifteen minutes you get to spend with that doctor a couple of times a year, all they can really do is give you advice. And as I'm sitting here writing this, I'm thinking back and realizing that while I'm really sure they meant well, and the things they were telling me were correct, it just didn't click. And I guess this is one of the most important parts of this book and my journey is that as a twelve-year-old kid, I asked myself how I could get to the finish line they were talking about. It was tough enough getting me to run that race that they hardly could get me motivated to even start! There has to be that special mixture of good information, just enough reality, and a whole lot of inspiration. And it's gonna have to come from within.

Let's take all this medical advice and use it to understand why I was feeling so lousy physically. Because if we don't start to change and feel better, it's very tough to move in the right direction. As the weight started to come off, my attitude started to change, my medical problems seemed to get much better, and all of the sudden my doctor's appointments became one of the highlights of my month, because I knew I was feeling better and I knew they could help me track my progress.

So here's the really cool thing about being a kid: making this lifestyle change is 100 percent easier now than it is when we get to be our parents' age. Time and youth are our biggest allies. Even if it's really tough to get started, it is so much easier now than it is later. Don't be afraid of the doctors. Don't be intimidated by the scales. Like everything else we are doing on our journey, use those things as resources. So the answer to, "What's up, Doc?" is our attitude, our outlook, and our future.

CHAPTER 4

Checkup from the Neck Up

A few days ago, Gang Greene got together to celebrate Kaila's and Granni's birthdays. Maybe you can guess what we did: we went out for a big family meal. (Some things never change—although what we order at these family meals sure has!)

I used to look forward to these family feasts so much that I actually dreamed about them, which, when I look back, is kind of scary. Then I met Dr. Craighead, who taught me a really simple thing that totally changed the way I eat. She taught me how to figure out when I was hungry, and when I wasn't.

I met Dr. Craighead the day I went on *The Dr. Oz Show*. We were getting into the elevator on our way up to do the show, and this lady stepped in with us. The next time I saw her was on national

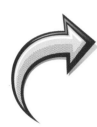

Linda W. Craighead, Ph.D.

I first met Tiger and his parents on *The Dr. Oz Show*. At lunch after the show, I realized right away that Mom and Dad were very motivated to help Tiger. Mom had already made a lot of changes in the family's meals, but I felt the family could use some help to make the changes feel more positive and to make sure that Tiger learned to make healthier choices on his own.

Parents have the essential job of making healthy food available and limiting exposure to unhealthy foods, but at twelve years old, Tiger (or any kid) had to learn how to manage his own appetite. If parents try to be the food police, the kid will not learn and may end up sneaking food. Parents can help their kids remember to use their Hunger Meter (explained below) and make the journey to health a family trip.

Tiger was amazing. He really listened and wanted to learn how he could lose weight. However, Tiger did love food, and he was used to eating large amounts.

The first lesson I taught Tiger was not to let himself get really hungry. Eat smaller amounts every three or four hours rather than waiting until you're starving, when you eat too fast and get stuffed. Second, stop eating when you feel just moderately full even though the food still tastes good. These are tough changes for kids to make, and Tiger couldn't make these changes all by himself. The whole family's lifestyle had to change to support him. It wasn't easy, but they did it!

> Dr. Linda Craighead received her Ph.D. from Pennsylvania State University in clinical psychology and is now a professor of psychology and director of the clinical psychology training program at Emory University in Atlanta. She developed a program called Appetite Awareness Training (AAT), described in her self-help manual called *The Appetite Awareness Workbook*. This was later adapted for families with overweight kids by Dr. Nancy L. Zucker at the Duke Center for Eating Disorders in Durham, North Carolina.

TV, after Dr. Oz had just told the world how close to death my dad and I were. She worked with my family for a pretty long time, helping us understand how Dad and I had gotten to this point and what it would take to change. This was no easy job. But she did it, I got it, and now she's willing to help me reach as many kids and families as we can together.

Anyway, Dr. Craighead taught me to recognize when I was hungry and when I was full. You might be thinking, *Who doesn't know when they're hungry or full?* Well, I didn't, and as it turns out, most big kids don't. Full is a funny concept to us! I don't know about you, but I ate all the time, whether I was hungry or not.

But things are different now. For our celebration, we went to this old Southern, home-style cooking restaurant Granni chose for the fresh veggies—yeah, right. This is the kind of place that serves fried this, smothered that, and pies the size of football helmets (don't give me a hard time—football season just started).

In the old days—I call them BC: Before Craighead—I'd have ordered fried appetizers *and* a slice of pie, and I would have convinced Dad to order a different slice so I could try that too. I'd order my entrée and eat that, and try everyone else's. I would eat until the food was gone or I just couldn't eat any more. And I wouldn't give one thought to how full I was even after the meal was over. I was used to that miserable, completely stuffed feeling after every meal!

But Dr. Craighead taught me to ask myself two questions before I ate anything, even one French fry:

1. How hungry am I?

2. Worth it or not worth it?

These questions are part of this cool idea Dr. Craighead taught me: the idea that everyone—me, you, your parents, your dog, your cat—has a built-in Hunger Meter that can tell you how hungry or full you are, on a scale of 1 (starving) to 5 (stuffed).

Starving	Hungry	Neutral	Satisfied	Stuffed
1	2 Start eating here	3	4 Stop eating here	5
Very, very hungry—too hungry! You may feel weak, your stomach may hurt, or you may have a headache.	Your stomach feels empty and may be growling. You are ready to eat!	You are not hungry but not yet satisfied!	You are not hungry and you may feel uncomfortable if you ate more.	You feel a little too full and feel uncomfortable.

The Appetite Awareness Workbook—Linda Craighead, Ph.D. (New Harbinger, 2006)
Courtesy of Linda Craighead, Ph.D., and Nancy Zucker, Ph.D.

My Hunger Meter

1. STARVING
   I'm totally starving. Lock up all small children and farm animals—I'm goin' on a rampage!

2. HUNGRY
   Haven't eaten in at least four hours and getting a little darn cranky. I gotta get me some groceries.

3. NEUTRAL
   My gas tank's pretty full. I'm not totally topped off, I've still got energy, and I'm ready to rock and roll.

4. SATISFIED
   Ugh. I'm a little slow to get up from the table. Stuffed is just a few bites away. Gotta head out for a walk.

5. STUFFED
   I can't believe I feel this bad again. I'm trading barbells and a jog for a joystick and a nap.

The Hunger Meter

Think of your Hunger Meter as the gas gauge on a car. The needle is on *F* when the tank is full and on *E* when it's empty. Everyone's Hunger Meter is kind of like that. Using my Hunger Meter made Kaila's and Granni's birthday dinner into a real celebration rather than the Foodapalooza it could have been.

Just before we left the house, I ate some fruit and drank a bottle of water to get me to 2 on the Hunger Meter. A 2 means you're a little hungry, but not starving.

So when Uncle Jeff and Uncle Larry ordered the appetizers for our table (grilled chicken wings stuffed with sausage—gross!), I passed on them. I wasn't so hungry I just had to have some no matter what. I was able to stop and think, *Is a few bites of greasy chicken really worth it?* Now I know what kind of food to order, and I was pretty content with just my entrée: lump crab cake with lots of crab and very little filler like bread crumbs (I asked before I ordered it), and sauce on the side. I also had my favorite veggies: black-eyed peas and collard greens. I only had a few bites of black-eyed peas so I could save room for cake. (Oh yeah—our server also gave us a big basket of cornbread and rolls. I didn't eat them. I bowled with them. You stack 'em like a pyramid and can knock 'em down with one roll if you hit it just right.)

I had such a great time hanging out with my family, I didn't focus on the food that much. That fruit and water I'd had earlier, and my entrée, filled me up. Even more important, I *knew* that. My stomach was satisfied, and I knew what satisfied felt like.

BC, I wouldn't have stopped eating if there was food left on my plate—or on anyone else's. That was before I started using the Hunger Meter. But that day, I stopped because I knew I'd had enough. More important, my brain and stomach knew it. The only thing I was full of when we got up from the table was pride. And it tasted awesome.

So Much Food, So Much Time

There's a saying that it takes a village to raise a child. If your community is anything like mine, it would be fair to say it takes a village to put a kid in size XXL. I don't know where you're reading this from, but where I live, in a five-mile radius, I count four schools, one library and fifty-eight restaurants. Seriously?

Chances are, unless you live way out in the country, you know what I mean. When you go out, you see doughnut shops, fast-food places and pizza joints, and restaurants on every corner. When you stay in and watch TV or surf the net, you see ads showing groups of happy people enjoying a meal at this restaurant or that restaurant—meals that would give a grizzly bear (or a Tiger) a bellyache.

I'm not saying you shouldn't enjoy a meal out with friends and family. I do it all the time, as you'll see in Chapter 6. I'm just saying that we can get delicious, high-fat, high-calorie garbage whenever we want it—whether we go out or have it delivered—and that commercials encourage us to eat at any hour and for any occasion. And believe me—I didn't need any encouragement from them.

Because of these two things—a lot of food nearby and a lot of advertising that promotes it—it's easy to lose sight of when you're hungry. It's also way too easy to eat a lot when you're not really hungry and to actually stop thinking about whether you're hungry. In fact, you might lose sight of when you're actually hungry and when you're not!

Dr. Craighead taught me that kids at a healthy weight generally eat when they're hungry and stop when they're satisfied. They don't usually eat until they're stuffed. That's part of the reason it's easier for them to stay at a healthy weight. They just naturally get the signals that their stomachs and brains send out that say, "Feed me," or "Stop eating." (Although I never really got that whole stop-eating signal. *My* signal was the restaurant closing or getting the *look* from Mom.) The trick is learning to recognize your stomach signals—and you can.

At our house, we have the Hunger Meter magnet that Dr. Craighead gave us on our refrigerator. It's a reminder to always be aware of how hungry—or how full—we're feeling before we open that refrigerator door. As I began to use this most excellent tool, I learned that there are three ways to make sure you use it to its full advantage.

Step 1:
Eat at the same times every day.

Eat at regular times so you don't feel too hungry before you eat. For most people, that means eating breakfast, lunch, and dinner and two snacks every day. On a typical day, my eating schedule looks something like this:

- Breakfast: 7 A.M.

- Mid-morning snack: 10 A.M.

- Lunch: Noon

- Mid-afternoon snack: 3 P.M.

- Dinner: 6 P.M.

You can start with this schedule to see if it works for you and adjust it if you need to. The only thing that matters is that you follow it the same way every day. That way, your body learns that you will feed it at regular times so it doesn't have to tell you to look for food all the time. Basically, you and your body get on the same page about when it's time to eat.

BC, I usually skipped breakfast unless I slept late and it became brunch. Lunch (usually with Dad) was always huge, and dinner was a few man-size portions as well. In between meals, I'd eat whatever was in sight until it was gone. There really was no thought about whether I felt hungry. It was pretty much a food-fest all the time. After I started my journey, one of the first realizations I came to was that all my days and events revolved around food. To regain my life from food, I had to break this cycle.

The first couple of weeks on my new eating schedule, I really had to time out my meals and watch my portions. I also had to force myself to eat the in-between meals. It took a week or so, but I finally got on schedule. For me, hunger is no longer an overwhelming, full-body I'm-gonna-die-if-I-don't-eat feeling because my schedule means there's always a little fuel in my tank. And when I run low, it's time for the next meal or snack. Now I know when I need to get some healthy food right away to prevent myself from getting too hungry and eating too much unhealthy food later. I still want food sometimes when I'm not really hungry, but now I think, *I could eat this snack or junk food, but do I want to work out an extra hour to burn it off?* Most of the time, I decide I don't. I'd rather be able to run faster, feel better, and live longer. Boy, times have changed.

Step 2:
Eat every three to four hours, at least.

Dr. Craighead recommended that every time I eat, I eat enough that I won't be hungry for at least three hours. Personally, I find eating every three to four hours works best for me, but you might want to start with the three-hour rule. You can adjust it according to what your Hunger Meter is telling you. One thing, though: a piece of fruit is healthy, but an apple or banana alone won't keep you satisfied for three hours. You actually have to eat a very small meal—enough to get you through those three hours. My favorite in-between snacks—the EnerZ wrap or hummus and whole-grain pita chips—are easy to wrap up and take

with you. In a pinch, fast-food places have some healthy offerings, which I talk about in Chapter 6.

After the first week or so of eating every three to four hours, your system becomes an alarm clock. I can bet you after your system gets used to knowing it's going to get what it needs on that schedule, you could hide all your watches and clocks and you would get hungry within that three- to four-hour window without fail. I can also promise if you stick with a schedule, you will never feel starved. If you aren't starving, it is easier not to overeat and it just doesn't seem worth it!

Step 3:
Use the Hunger Meter
every time you want to eat.

You will learn pretty quickly how each number on the Hunger Meter feels to you, and you probably already know how 1 and 5 feel. To keep from getting to those numbers, your job is to avoid feeling starved before you eat. If you stay away from 1, you are less likely to eat to 5!

Let's say you're at the mall and you just ate your scheduled meal an hour and a half ago. You see the pizza place. I'll bet you will find that although you might *want* a slice of pizza, a quick check of your Hunger Meter will show you that you aren't truly hungry. Most of the time, you'll find that you get hungry at about the same time you have a scheduled meal. If you think you are hungry before it's time for a scheduled meal, trust me—you are probably just bored. When it comes to food, boredom can be one of your worst enemies.

There's no one right way to use the Hunger Meter. I know how I feel when I'm stuffed, starving, or neutral, but my 5, 1, and 3 are likely different from yours. Each of us has to listen to and learn from our own body. That's part of the journey, and it's kind of cool to decode your body's hunger signals for yourself!

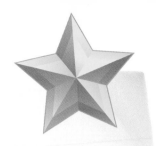

Sarah's Story

One Saturday I was at the Little League park, staffing a small grill behind my grandma's concession stand. As I turned chicken breasts for my Team Tiger Healthier Choice menu, I heard my grandma say, "Yes, he's here. He's out back." A second later, a girl my age came around the side of the stand and gave me a big hug. "Thank you for everything," she said.

I recognized her from school—her name was Sarah. Her mom came over a few minutes later to explain what I'd done to deserve such a sweet and heartfelt hug.

Sarah is autistic, her mom explained. Sarah wasn't big, but she'd seen me on TV and had decided to change her diet. Like me before my journey, Sarah tended toward junk food, but seeing and hearing my story motivated her to follow my example.

As Sarah's diet changed—from candy, cheeseburgers, and fries to fruit, veggies, and grilled chicken—Sarah's mother noticed that Sarah seemed calmer and more focused, and she was doing better in school. Sarah and her mom also started walking during her brother's Little League games instead of just heading to Grandma's concession stand. (Grandma wasn't thrilled with that part.)

Sarah's mom told me that although she had taken Sarah to many specialists, it wasn't until she changed her eating and exercise habits that things turned around. A healthier, more active lifestyle can do more than change your weight. It can change your life.

"Worth It or Not Worth It?"

After Dr. Oz's show, when Dr. Craighead started working with my family, she kept saying that we were all in this healthy lifestyle change together. One of the first things she taught us was to think through our food choices with the phrase "Worth it or not worth it?"

When I heard this, I was pretty sure it was a silly idea and that there was no way that this question would stand between me and a milkshake.

But a few days later, Dad was in his office working, and I was in mine doing homework. Dad was having a tough day—he was on call after call, and he kept grabbing his head in his hands. At some point, he came to my door and told me he was going to the bank. I got up to go with him, but he waved me back to my seat. "Stay with the guys. I'll be right back," he said.

I thought this was kind of strange—he loves having us kids with him all the time, even if he's just running errands. But he looked so stressed, I didn't push it.

About twenty minutes later, my phone rang. It was Dad, sounding a little weird. "I'm at the drive-through at McDonald's," he said. "I got this craving for a Big Mac meal, a Filet-O-Fish, and a Coke." (This was his standing order at Mickey D's.) "How do you fight off these cravings now?"

To my surprise, I said, "Is that food worth it?" It was the first time I'd thought about this "silly" phrase since Dr. Craighead told us about it. Now, it didn't seem so dumb.

"Is it worth another heart surgery and me possibly losing you?" I continued. (Ah, young grasshopper—the student becomes the teacher.)

He didn't say anything, so I added, "If you're really craving a burger, then let's go get a lean burger with no bun. That can be our next meal."

After another pause, he told me he loved me and would be back at the office shortly. When he got back, I gave him a big hug and kiss. (I wanted to see if he smelled like fries. Sorry to ruin the moment.) He passed the test and all of us ask that silly question to ourselves and each other pretty often, even today.

Get to 4 and No More

To be honest with you, I think the description of 5 on the Hunger Meter is a little inaccurate. You feel a *little* too full? You feel *uncomfortable?*

I don't know about you, but to me, *stuffed* means I've eaten to the point where I actually feel sick to my stomach. I know that feeling well—by the time I started my journey, I had been at 5 on the Meter after 99 percent of the meals I'd eaten in my lifetime. I always thought, *Why would you stop when there is still food around?* Now I know why you have to decide for yourself when you need to stop eating.

So here's the big question: How do you know when you are a 4 on the Hunger Meter, and how do you stop there? If you eat like I used to, you feel like you're at 5 after most meals and you have no idea how you got there!

Here's how I do it. I eat more slowly now. Sometimes I put my fork down between bites. Or I do a lot more talking than eating. I used to eat with my head down because I thought everyone was watching the big kid pig out. Now, I use meals as an opportunity to catch up as well as fuel up. I want people to see what's on Tiger's plate (as you will in Chapter 5). I keep paying attention to how my stomach feels as I eat. And as soon as I feel like I'm not hungry anymore, I stop.

When I stop eating, I feel good. My stomach feels good. I don't feel like I have to take a nap after I eat. Basically, I feel energized and alert—like I could go for a walk. (And sometimes I do.)

I've learned that it doesn't take as much food as I thought to get that satisfied feeling. Dr. Craighead told me that your empty stomach is just a little bigger than the size of your fist. Your stomach stretches so you can eat more than that, but every time you overeat, your stomach

forgets that it doesn't need all that food to feel satisfied. You kind of have to train it. It will take maybe a week for your stomach to feel satisfied with less food and to start signaling you: "Okay, that's enough. I could eat more, but I don't need more."

And hey, I can always eat again in three hours. So get to 4 and no more. Your stomach will thank you.

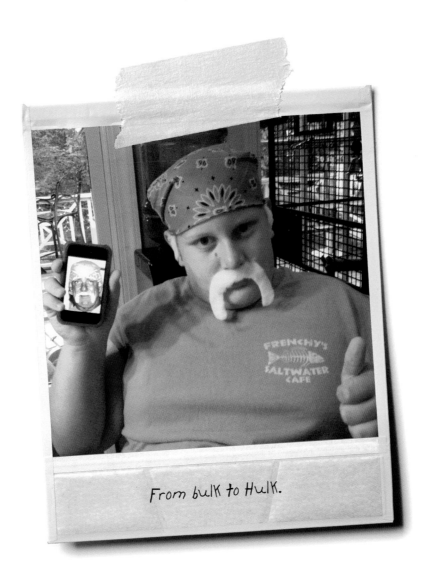

From bulk to Hulk.

Chalk Talk with My Dad:
How Parents Can Help

Of all the guidelines, creating and sticking to an eating schedule can be the toughest on parents, especially if you're not living or eating quite as healthy as you'd like. (Believe me, I've been there.) Dr. Craighead told us that we wouldn't change lifelong habits overnight. But we found that it was much easier when our whole family adopted healthier eating habits together.

A few days before we started, we sat down and brainstormed healthy snacks and meals we all liked. We also wrote out a shopping list together and did a group trip to the grocery store, where we read food labels and discussed our choices.

We began our schedule on a Saturday morning and chose to eat three small meals and two good-size snacks a day. Make meals and snacks smaller than those you eat now but large enough to satisfy you for at least three or four hours. We give you lots of great meal and snack ideas in Chapter 5.

If you eat out a lot, plan a few restaurant meals so everyone in your family experiences what it's like to eat smaller portions and make healthier choices at their favorite restaurants. (You'll find tips on dining out in Chapter 6.)

Throughout the weekend, at every meal or snack, we compared notes using the Hunger Meter. "So we ate three hours ago. Are you at 1, 2, or 3? What does 1, 2, or 3 feel like? Do we like eating every three hours, or should we try eating every four hours instead?" Talking in Hunger Meter language helped everyone understand the difference between being truly hungry and having a craving.

After that first weekend, we just kept going. We planned dinner around our family's eating schedule. Before and after dinner, we compared notes on where we fell on the Hunger Meter. Above all, we stuck to our schedule, no matter how hectic life got.

(Don't say your week is too hectic. You haven't lived with us!)

We also made sure we stocked healthy snacks at home, and packed them for school too. You may want to schedule a school conference, as we did, so teachers and the principal understand what you're doing and why your child needs to eat a snack each school day at, say, two P.M. After a week or two, our new schedule became a part of our lifestyle.

Once we changed our eating habits as a family, it was easier for Tiger to succeed. You might find yourself succeeding right along with your child. This journey isn't just about our kids. It's about our families, our communities, and our future. And it's never too late to change. I'm living proof.

One of My Many 5 Stories

Okay, you now know what 5 on the Hunger Meter means. It means you're totally *stuffed*. This is one of my many, many "I Got to 5!" stories—and let me tell you, I never want to relive another one!

Did you ever watch that show called *Man v. Food* on the Travel Channel? Well, for one episode, the host of the show went to Atlanta. He visited two restaurants. One was Gladys Knight's Chicken and Waffles, and the other was Big Pie in the Sky Pizzeria, this pizza place that does something called the Carnivore Challenge. The challenge: two people have to eat one of their pizzas in one hour.

This is not just any pizza. When you do the challenge, you get a pizza that *weighs eleven pounds,* five pounds of which are meat toppings. The people on the show who'd accepted the challenge gave up halfway through and actually lost their lunch (or dinner).

After we saw that show, but before my journey began, my family (okay, Dad and I) decided to have our own Man v. Food weekend. (Yes, just a little different from running a 5K and then hitting the farmers' market.)

So one Saturday afternoon we drove twenty-eight miles to Atlanta for fried chicken and waffles. Dad and I ordered—and finished—two entrées each and several appetizers. Kaila, Zack, and Mom could only manage one entrée each (those lightweights!).

After this, my mom and Kaila threw in the towel. So the next day, Dad, Zack, and I headed forty miles to Big Pie in the Sky. We were gonna take that pizza *down*.

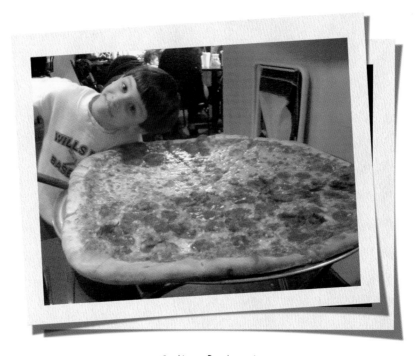

Golden Rule #1:
Never eat anything bigger than your brother.

We sat down, ordered sodas (I was still drinking regular Coke then), and waited an hour for them to make this behemoth pizza. We actually had appetizers while we were waiting.

They finally brought this eleven-pound pizza to our table. No lie, it was the size of one of those snow saucers you use to sled down hills. Dad and I only managed one slice each, one slice equaling roughly half a normal pizza. Somehow—I still can't believe it—my skinny little brother managed to eat *two* slices. (He was very proud and pronounced himself a true Greene.) Each slice was bigger than he was.

Dad and I couldn't believe we'd failed the challenge, but we felt too sick to care. We rolled out of the place, crawled into the car, totally miserable, and moaned all the way home.

I never forgot how awful I felt. In fact, when I started my journey and felt a little hungry after a meal, I'd remember that exact misery and swear that I'd never feel it again. All of a sudden, that second helping of dessert didn't seem so appetizing.

Everybody's Got a Hungry Heart

I know that all of this checkup-from-the-neck-up stuff can be a little scary and/or boring. And I was so sick of people telling me I was eating because I was bored or eating because I was depressed or to stop eating even when the food was awesome. But it was really helpful for me to understand what was going on and why. I'm not as dumb as I look (please don't ask Kaila for her opinion on that), so when I decided to change my life, I had to understand what I was changing. Hang in here with me—this is important stuff.

If you eat for any reason other than to satisfy physical hunger, you might be using food to deal with your feelings. You might hit the chips or cookies hard when you're stressed out, sad, lonely, or angry. But being happy might also cause you to eat—like when you reward yourself for a good report card or other achievement. My number-one food downfall is celebrating good times.

Even people who are at a healthy weight eat emotionally at times. I mean, why do people go out for ice cream on a summer night? Because they're happy—it's summer, they're with friends, and ice cream happens to rock. (So does nonfat yogurt, my favorite! Unless it's yogurt with 10 million calories' worth of unhealthy toppings.) But for some people, emotional eating is a problem. The biggest thing to know about it is that when you do it, you're not really hungry. Don't roll your eyes—I'm serious. It's just that somehow, you figured out that when you eat the foods you love, really love, you feel better.

Until you swallow the last bite. The pleasure of eating ends when you finish the ice cream, but you'll still be stressed out, lonely, angry, or bored (not to mention sick to your stomach). You might also feel bad about eating the amount or type of food you did. My dad calls it the buyer's remorse of the food chain.

For help, turn to your Hunger Meter. It's the first step to figuring out whether your body actually needs food or if you're just looking for comfort.

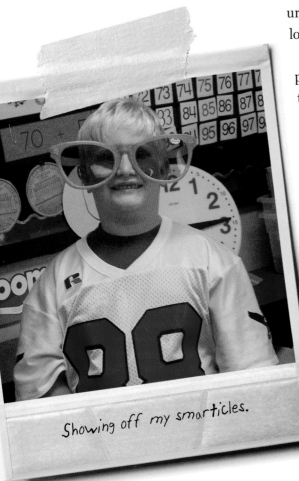

Showing off my smarticles.

CHAPTER 5

Eat like a Tiger!

Being the food lovers we are, Dad and I do a lot of the grocery shopping. After we ask the family what they want and add it to our list, we head to our local Publix, where everyone knows us. Once inside, we head straight for the cooking demonstration. We always stop to see what's cooking and usually try it.

A few days ago, the cook made two dishes—Tuscan-style chicken and sautéed white beans. One of the things I've learned about nutrition is that the more colorful the plate, the healthier and more appealing it usually is, and this was a meal with color! The chicken included spinach and tomatoes, and the white beans were made with roasted red peppers. The cook also made a salad, and the whole meal looked like a delicious rainbow. I grabbed the recipe card and ingredients—the store has them all right there for you. I knew what we'd be having for dinner the next night.

Then we hit the deli section. I like being the one to pick out the deli meats and plan what I'll be taking to school for lunch for the next few days. Next,

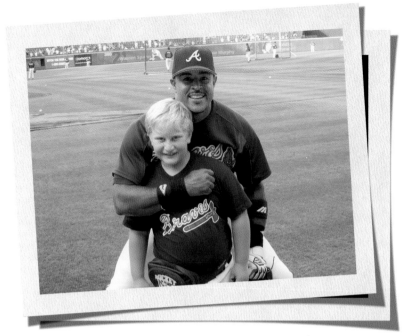

I've met so many great people on my journey.
This is me with Atlanta Braves' Brian Jordan.

we wheeled our cart over to the ammo depot—I mean, the produce section. When I said everyone at our Publix knows us, it's not necessarily because they've seen me on TV. Did you know the fruit that is closest in size to a football is a cantaloupe? If I'm in the store, most of the customers do. They also know that lemons and limes are great for juggling.

I didn't always cruise the aisles of the supermarket, especially not the outer aisles, where the healthy foods tend to be. But since then I've learned a little about nutrition, and now it's cool to have a say on what foods make it into our refrigerator and pantry and end up on our plates. Even better, as I was learning to eat healthier, my little brother and sister learned right along with me. Now, wherever we are, Kaila, Zack, and I always know what kinds of foods should be on our plates to keep us healthy. One of the most important things we learned is that it's okay not to like some foods. For example, I will never, ever like brussels sprouts. But it's cool to at least try everything.

At school one day after I started my journey, I told one of my favorite teachers about how I'd gotten into going to Publix with my dad. Her face lit up (which kind of startled me—who would have guessed she'd get so excited about grocery shopping?), and she said I had to meet her friend, nutritionist Kim Wilson ("Mrs. Kim"). After we met, I knew we needed her to help us at the Georgia Dome. Mrs. Kim made learning about nutrition fun for the kids—she compared their bodies to Ferraris and healthy foods to premium fuel—and I learned a few things myself.

If you're willing to learn a super small amount about nutrition—the absolute least you need to know—you're reading the right book! The upcoming pictures tell you pretty much everything you need to know:

Meet the Team Tiger Expert!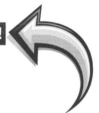

Kim Wilson, NCCPT

When I met Tiger, I was impressed by his passion to teach every young person he meets what he's learned about how to get and stay healthy. He's absolutely committed to helping them, and their families, to get the information and help they need to live healthier, happier lives. Team Tiger, which brings together professionals who have this information with the kids and families who need it—in a way that's simple and fun—is both genius and common sense.

It's imperative that we teach young people the fundamentals of wellness, like a healthy diet and regular exercise. Tiger is taking his personal journey to the streets, so to speak, and building a major movement in the fight against childhood obesity. I was honored to spend time with a young man so full of life and so committed to helping others.

Kim Wilson is a certified personal trainer, certified weight-management specialist, and fitness/nutrition coach to more than fifty young athletes at the Alpharetta Tennis Academy, which she owns with her husband, Jeff, a professional tennis coach, in Alpharetta, Georgia. They have three children. She serves as trainer and fitness/nutrition coach to Irina Falconi, currently one of the highest-ranked U.S. female tennis players by the Women's Tennis Association.

Eat every three to four hours, and definitely eat breakfast.

When you eat, watch your portion sizes.

Whether you're eating breakfast, lunch, dinner, or a snack, make what's on your plate look like mine. This is one instance where it's okay to copy off someone else! No, you don't need to eat *exactly* what's on my plate—you'll have a lot more choices than you think.

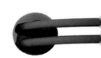

Breakfast:
Don't Blow It Off

To be honest, breakfast isn't one of my favorite meals—I have to force myself to eat it. But I do it because I've learned that to get my motor running, I need to get some of that premium fuel into me within an hour of waking up.

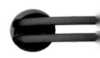

Breakfast used to be several bagels with cream cheese, or those fast-food breakfast sandwiches (like most of you, I'm always on the go). No more—grease isn't the best fuel you can put in your tank, and those itty-bitty breakfast sandwiches contain a ton of calories.

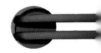

Now, my favorite breakfast is an EnerZ wrap—I spread a whole-wheat tortilla with one tablespoon of peanut butter, top it with a sliced banana, sprinkle on a little granola for crunch, add some raisins and a little honey or agave nectar, and roll it up. My next favorite: a whole-grain English muffin with peanut butter or the best sausage links ever—they are actually soy sausages, made by Morningstar Farms. Or I might have an egg-white omelet with whole-grain toast and fruit, or fruit with yogurt. I wash it all down with a glass of 1% milk, then a glass of water. I don't drink juice too often—it has a lot of sugar in it, so it's one of my treats.

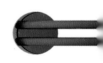

It can be tough to find really healthy fast-food breakfast options, so I try to eat breakfast at home before we get movin'. Because once we are out and about—game on!

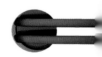

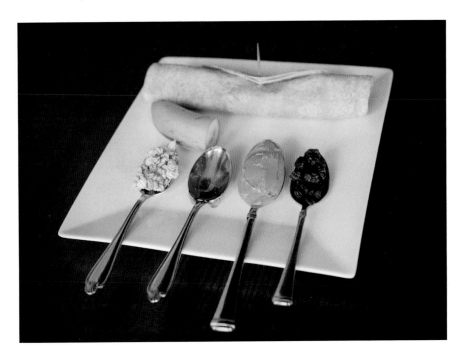

EnerZ wrap.

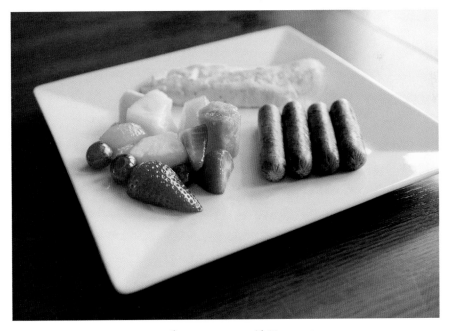

Soy sausage links.

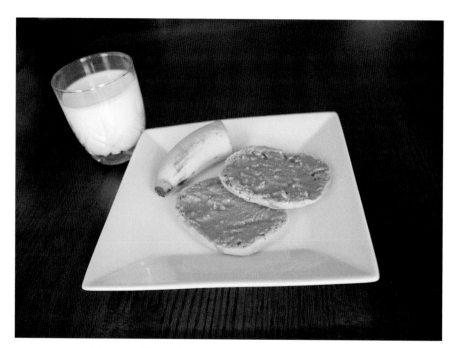

English muffin with light coat of peanut butter.

How Much Food Do **You** Need?

Mrs. Kim told me that how much kids need to eat is based on stuff like how old they are, whether they're a boy or a girl, and how active they are. Just as an example, my eleven-year-old sister, Kaila, who gets at least some moderate exercise every day, needs more food than a moderately active seven-year-old, and boys generally need a couple hundred more calories a day than girls if their activity levels are similar. And of course, an active kid (who's playing a sport or who gets an hour or more of moderate to vigorous activity a day) needs more food than a kid who gets only thirty minutes of normal activity a day.

This is where your parents, or maybe your doctor, come into the picture. They can tell you exactly how much food you need. If you're really interested (or if your parents are), tell them to check out www.choose myplate.gov, which lets you customize a daily menu especially for you.

Lunch: Tigerize It!

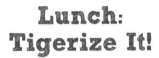

If you're like most kids, you can pack lunch or buy it at school. The good news is, most school cafeterias have at least some healthy options. You may have to develop an eagle eye (or eye of the Tiger) to pick them out, but the more you do it, the better at it you'll get.

At first, the best way to choose the healthy options is to read the cafeteria menu. Most schools list it on their websites (print it out every week), and some schools send home an entire month of menus. Figure out the healthy options for each day—your parents can help with this. When you've found them, circle them—and stick to them. Then you'll automatically know what's on *your* menu every day.

At school, I usually choose one of the salads they offer with dressing on the side, or a chicken or turkey wrap. I add either yogurt or fresh fruit. No more sugary sodas or fruit juice for me either—just a bottle or two of water. That lunch brings me to a 4 on my Hunger Meter, and I can get on with the rest of my day without falling asleep in class.

Even if you choose healthy options, the school lunch staff will probably give you huge amounts, so use your palm to figure out how much of anything to eat. I always choose a palm-size portion of protein—chicken, fish, or meat—along with veggies and a palm-size portion of starches or grains. Try to choose whole grains, like whole-wheat bread or brown rice, but if your school doesn't offer them, opt for a piece of fruit or a low-fat yogurt, if they are available. If it's pizza or taco day, treat yourself to one slice or one taco along with a salad, light dressing on the side. (Sometimes I put some of the salad on the pizza or in the taco. It's pretty good—try it!)

If you take lunch to school, you'll usually get a healthier meal and you're guaranteed to get the healthy stuff you like rather than what the cafeteria is offering that day. Of course, you've got to pack healthy options rather than chips and cookies. If you take lunch to school, check out pages 97–98—you'll find lots of healthy take-from-home lunches.

If you want to pack your lunch, ask your parents to help. Talk to them about what you like to eat for lunch, and then go shopping with them! (Check out the shopping lists on pages 110–12—they can get you started.)

For me, eating smaller portions was the biggest lunchtime change. Once I started eating breakfast and a small mid-morning snack, downsizing my lunch became pretty easy. In the school lunch line, I was at a 3 on the Hunger Meter and could make healthier choices and eat healthy amounts.

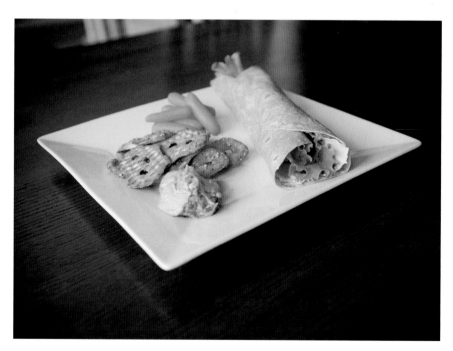

Ham and lettuce.

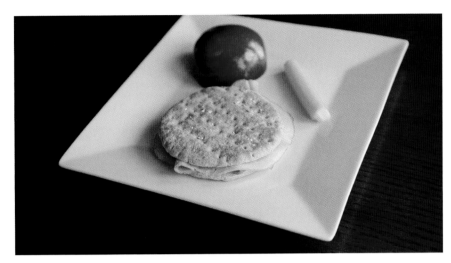

Turkey sandwich.

Sack the Boring Bag Lunch!

If you bring your lunch to school, it's easy to get bored with taking the same old thing and go back to the often-unhealthy cafeteria or vending-machine stuff. But if you and your family put together a weekly plan, shop together, and have fun in the kitchen, you can bring bag lunches that are not only healthy but also contain food that you actually like.

I like to use flatbread or whole-wheat tortilla wraps, with turkey, all-white tuna, lean roast beef, or lean, low-sodium ham. Then I add grapes or other fresh fruit (no prepackaged fruit cups loaded with syrup), wheat pita chips or a single-serving bag of popcorn, and usually a low-fat yogurt or string cheese. I also add veggies: baby carrots, celery with a teaspoon of peanut butter, or cucumber slices with the same amount of light ranch dressing or salsa. Whatever I don't eat, I keep as a snack for later.

Or, when your mom or dad cooks a healthy dinner or you go out to eat and have leftovers (of course, you made healthy choices!), have it again for lunch the next day. To keep it warm, you or your parents can heat it up in the morning before school and then pack it in one of those insulated containers.

I also like to do theme days of the week. There's Mexican Monday with a tortilla wrap using rotisserie or grilled chicken and salsa. To make my friends laugh, sometimes I take an extra wrap, make a mask, and become Tortilla Libre. (Really, I do. You aren't surprised at this point, are you?) Then there's Turkey Tuesday, when I do a turkey sandwich loaded with lettuce, mustard, and tomato, or chili made with ground turkey, or roasted turkey breast that my dad makes with lemon pepper seasoning. I'll leave it to you to be creative on the rest of the days, but you could always do Fun Friday, which is my favorite. I might have a homemade mini pizza made with a whole-wheat sandwich round (we call it a Zackaroni pizza—see recipe below), a homemade sub (with the inside of the roll scooped out), or my Team Tiger Chicken Sandwich (the kind we sell at my grandma's concession stand) with a little honey Dijon mustard.

Zackaroni Pizza

If it's time for lunch or dinner and you're dying for pizza, try the kind Zack "invented." It really hits the spot, but it won't leave you feeling stuffed.

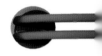

    1 whole-wheat sandwich round
    A couple tablespoons of jarred pizza sauce—
        the low-fat, low-sodium kind
    A couple tablespoons of 1% mozzarella cheese
        (the shredded kind in the bag)
    Mini turkey pepperoni

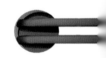

Open sandwich round and lay flat, add on sauce, top with the cheese and pepperoni, and then stick the round in your toaster oven or microwave until the cheese melts. (Zack likes twenty-one seconds in the microwave 'cause that's his football number—I like using the toaster oven so it's crispier.) Presto—pizza!

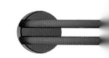

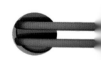

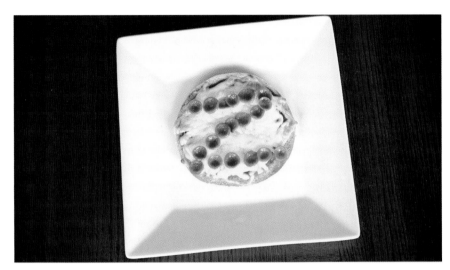

Zackaroni pizza.

Dinner:
Food <u>and</u> Family Time

Before I started my journey, dinner used to be the highlight of my family's day. In fact, we would often plan our days around our meals, especially dinner, and we allowed plenty of time for our nightly feast. Dinner is still the highlight of our day, but for totally different reasons.

Now we plan and make healthy dinners as a family, and it's a lot of fun. Sometimes, one of us gets to choose the entire meal that day; other times, we each choose one part of the meal and then go to the supermarket or farmers' market together to pick everything out. An hour or so before dinner, we crank up the music and get it ready together.

Even though we are family, it's easy to see the difference in taste from our choices. I'm usually a meat and potatoes (well, now a half potato) guy, Kaila would be content with just fruit, and Zack likes Zackaroni pizza or some strange combo sandwich that always tastes better than it looks. But there are a few meals that we all love and that are often on our table.

Spaghetti—we serve whole-wheat pasta and make a homemade sauce with lean ground sirloin or turkey breast. We add lots of veggies to the sauce too.

Grilled chicken—marinated in light Italian dressing with lemon pepper seasoning, served with salad.

Turkey burgers—made with ground turkey breast (we eat them with whole-wheat buns or sometimes no buns at all), served with pita chips and hummus or blue chips with salsa and a veggie— maybe my dad's garlic broccoli. He sautés the broccoli in light virgin olive oil until it's kind of tender but still crisp and then tosses in fresh chopped or minced garlic until it turns brown. (I add a little crushed pepper to Tiger it up.) He also stir-fries asparagus with a pinch of kosher salt and ground pepper in light virgin olive oil—it's ready quick, and we all love it.

Steak—(a lean cut) served with grilled squash and zucchini (my favorite!) and half a baked potato with a teaspoon of margarine and a dash of pepper.

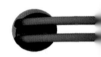

Salmon—pan-seared, served with asparagus and grilled tomatoes, seasoned with lemon pepper and topped with a pinch of Italian-style bread crumbs and Parmesan cheese.

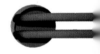

One of our most fun meals is kebab night, when Mom and Dad grill a bunch of different veggies (green, red, and yellow bell peppers, sweet Vidalia onions, cherry tomatoes, mushrooms) and cut-up steak and chicken and we all get to make our own kebabs (the most colorful one wins). With a salad or Dad's famous garlic broccoli, we have a touchdown!

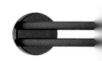

Maybe you have noticed that we eat a lot of lean beef, chicken, and fish and veggies. But Zack and Mike love pasta and Kaila loves mashed potatoes, so we do eat some starches, and you can too if you serve yourself a palm-size portion. Take it from me—when you have a balanced plate, a little starch goes a long way and you'll leave the table feeling satisfied, not stuffed.

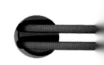

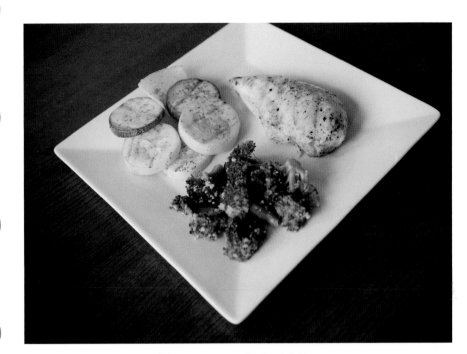

Six-ounce grilled chicken.

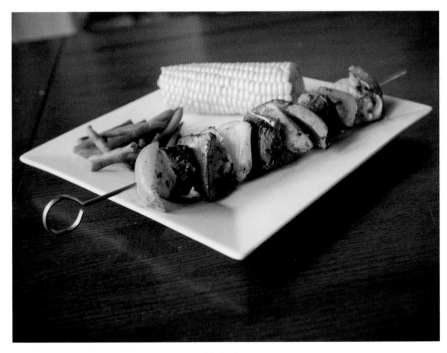

Kebabs.

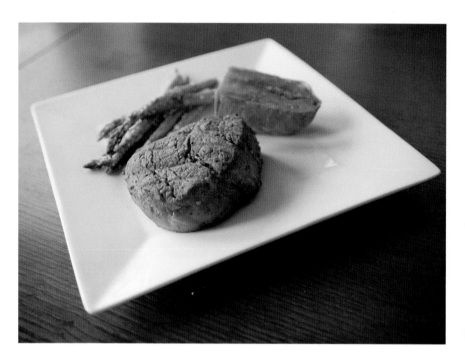

One eight-ounce steak, 1/2 sweet potato, grilled asparagus.

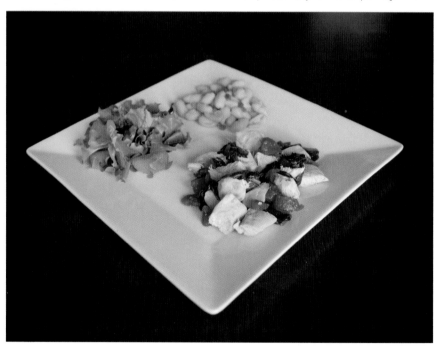

Tuscan chicken, white beans, salad.

Snacks:
Keep Your Motor Running!

Snack is a funny word to me. When I used to wipe out whole bags of chips or candy at a time—more calories than most people's dinners—and I was constantly eating between meals without much of a break, was I really snacking? I was always really good at eating—if it was a sport, I could have made the Olympics—and to me, *snacking* meant "not eating a meal," so I thought I could have as much as I wanted.

Wow, I didn't mean to rant. But snacks are such a different idea for me now. Just because they're smaller than meals doesn't mean they're not as important. Not only do small snacks maintain your energy and remind your body that it will get fed every few hours, but they also keep you from reaching a 1 on your Hunger Meter and then overeating.

So now, when my body is running low on high-test fuel, I top off the tank. All you'll find in my house to snack on now is fresh fruit, trail mix, yogurt, string cheese, hummus, celery and carrots, and protein shake mixes. (Actually, that's a lot of options.) When that between-meals belly alarm goes off, I reach for one of those. I add lowfat milk, water, or my favorite Powerade Zero, and life is good.

Because we're on the go all the time, our snacks travel with us. Dad keeps hummus and pita chips in his office refrigerator, and Mom brings trail mix and fresh fruit when we head out to wherever, and we always have a few granola bars in the car in case we're out all day. If you're always on the run too, you can do the same thing. For example, you might keep a healthy snack in your book bag to eat between classes or to hold you over if you have a long bus ride home and dinner is a few hours away.

I cannot put into words how good I feel compared to the old days except to say that I feel *so* good that I had to write this book to share what I've learned with you. Trust me—you'll love the feeling of being full of life rather than full of food, and smart snacking can help you do it!

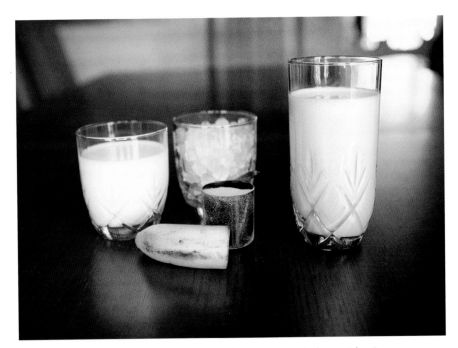

Chocolate banana protein shake, and ingredients

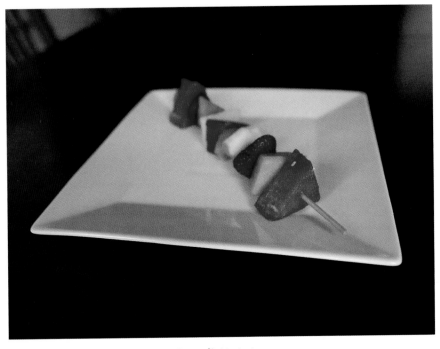

Fruit Kebabs.

Special Occasions: Celebrate the Event, Not the Meal

Gang Greene firmly believes that life is a celebration, and since I began my journey, I've never felt deprived or left out when it comes to holidays, birthday parties, or any other special occasion. Now I have learned to celebrate the event, not the meal.

If I am at school or at a party and they serve cake or hand out cupcakes, I can join in. I have a thin slice of cake or cut the cupcake in half depending on how sweet and how big it is. (And sometimes I eat the whole cupcake—how's that for a rebel?) But that's it—I don't go back for seconds. I don't chow down, either—I take small bites and make it last, which sometimes makes me not want the rest. Those treats really do taste way too sweet these days, and I have lost that loving feeling for them.

But most important at these events is to make your friends and family the focus of your celebration. The meal is just the fuel for you to enjoy the good stuff.

Chalk Talk with My Dad: How Parents Can Help

When it comes to nutrition, the biggest help we can be to our children is to remove temptation until they learn to make healthier choices on their own (and they will). In our house, removing temptation meant changing what we bought at the grocery store and—at first—fixing plates for the kids instead of letting them fix their own plates. Now I'm happy to say that every one of my kids knows exactly what should be on their plates to keep them healthy and fit.

Toss out the junk. The chips, the soda, the doughnuts, the processed pizzas, and boxed mac and cheese . . . get rid of it. ➔

Make a list and stick to it.   Until our new way of eating became a habit—and I learned to stick to the perimeter of the store—I found myself automatically grabbing chips and soda. Until "shopping on the edge" becomes second nature to you, use the list in this chapter. Eventually, you'll know exactly what your family likes—and so will your family.

Make shopping trips a family affair.   Pile the family in the car and make a group trip to the supermarket. It may take longer, but remember, you've got that list. Plus, it's a great way to get your whole family interested in trying out a fruit or vegetable you haven't tried before or taking a chance on a cool-sounding whole grain you saw in the organic section.

Make healthy snacks visible and accessible.   Cut up fruits and veggies and arrange them in the refrigerator at eye level. Keep the low-fat yogurt, string cheese, and single-serving bags of microwave popcorn stocked. In other words, make it a no-brainer for your children to grab a healthy snack.

Plan healthy meals together.   Look at the photos in this chapter and then make your children's plates look like them—you'll automatically improve your children's diet without thinking of protein, carbs, vitamins, or any other term out of a nutrition textbook. If your children are still hungry twenty minutes after their last bite, offer veggies or fruit.

Serve water with your meals.   It's not like the kids don't like their Powerade Zero or Marsha and I don't like our Arizona Diet Blueberry Iced Tea. But early on, we decided that water would be our primary beverage—our bodies need it, and it's the best thirst-quencher there is.

Remember: your children aren't on a diet. *Your family is eating healthier.* You are shopping differently, cooking differently, and thinking about nutrition differently. Don't say you can't do it. If you cared enough to buy this book, you can. We did.

A Note from Mrs. Kim:
"Dear Parents . . ."

I know how confusing nutrition information can be, and I won't confuse you any more than I need to! These tips can help you make sure your children are getting the nutrition they need as they lose weight and get healthier.

No matter how heavy your children are, they need to eat enough calories to support their growth and development. Ask your children's pediatrician to guide you. Make sure your children's menu contains lots of different types of foods so they will get enough protein, carbohydrates, fats, and vitamins and minerals.

- As much as possible, swap processed foods for whole foods—fruits and veggies, whole grains, meat, low-fat dairy. This will minimize your children's intake of saturated fat, trans fat, cholesterol, salt (sodium), and added sugars.
- Most of the fats in your children's diet should come from fish and plant foods, like nuts or nut butters and olive or canola oils.
- Serve whole-grain, high-fiber breads and cereals rather than refined grain products. Look for a whole grain as the first ingredient on the food label and make at least half your grain servings whole-grain.
- Serve a variety of fruits and vegetables daily while limiting juice intake. Each meal should contain at least one fruit or vegetable.
- Introduce and regularly serve fish as an entrée. Avoid commercially fried fish.
- Serve fat-free and low-fat dairy foods in appropriate serving sizes. From age one to eight, children need two cups of milk or its equivalent each day; ages nine and up, they need three cups. ➔

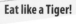

Need help managing your child's portion sizes? Try these simple tips:

- Offer a single serving of the main course of any meals you prepare at home and let your kids have extra salad or other vegetables if they are still hungry.

- If you want to cook in bulk to save time during the week, refrigerate or freeze individual-size portions so that your child will know how much to have.

- Choose child portions, small orders, or half orders for your child when you eat out at restaurants.

- Buy only single-serving or bite-size snacks.

- Review the label and repackage foods into single serving sizes. If a bag of cookies says that a single serving is three cookies, then put three cookies in a zippered plastic bag or on a plate when you give it to your kids.

- Avoid letting your kids just eat from a bag of snacks or a carton of ice cream—they will likely eat much more than one serving.

Super Tips for Super Shopping

When I hit the supermarket with my mom or dad, we always know what we need and where it is—and we know how to avoid temptation too.

Shop on the edge. Think about how your supermarket is laid out. Picture the sections along the outer edges of the store. What do you see? The produce section, where you find fruit, veggies, the salad bar, and prepared foods like rotisserie chicken. The deli section, where the lean lunch meats are. The meat and fish sections. The dairy section, where you pick up milk, cheese, yogurt, and eggs. The breads are usually near the dairy section.

The inner aisles contain most of the processed foods including soda, candy, and snack foods. You'll need to go to some inner aisles to pick up healthy stuff like canned beans, natural peanut butter, and high-fiber cereal, but get in and out of those aisles fast so you're not tempted by the junk food!

One more thing: the frozen-food section is generally one aisle away from the dairy section. Frozen fruit and veggies are just as healthy as fresh are as long as they don't include cheese and butter sauces. So if they're on your list, get them fast, and speed by the frozen French fries, garlic bread, ice cream, and the other not-so-healthy stuff.

Don't shop when you're hungry. Shopping on an empty stomach makes food look more tempting.

Make a list. Lists have become a big part of my journey—I have a list of goals I want to accomplish, a list of ways Team Tiger can reach and help other kids, and even a list of all the things I never thought I could do and the people who felt the same. This list—a shopping list—is my blueprint for successful nutrition. One of my friends in the NFL says if you stay ready, you don't have to get ready—having great options at home is staying ready.

Our Team Tiger shopping list (on the following pages) is based on the shopping-on-the-edge principle. All you need to do is photocopy this list, check the items you like and/or need, and go. Before long, you'll automatically stick to the edges of the store, with occasional quick trips into the inner aisles to restock cereals, pastas, and cooking oils.

Copy This Shopping List!

Fruit

❏ Fresh whole fruit (apples, oranges, pears, bananas, grapes)

❏ Berries (strawberries, blueberries, blackberries)

❏ Melon (cantaloupe, honeydew, watermelon)

❏ Tropical fruits (pineapple, mango, papaya, kiwi)

❏ Canned fruit (packed in 100% juice or light syrup)

Vegetables

❏ Dark leafy green: spinach, romaine, collards

❏ Dark green: avocados, broccoli, green bell peppers, asparagus, green beans

❏ Dark orange/yellow: butternut and acorn squash, yellow squash, carrots, sweet potatoes

❏ Red: tomatoes, red peppers

❏ Starchy: potatoes, corn on the cob

❏ Canned vegetables (packed in low-salt water and drained before you cook them)

Meat, poultry, and seafood

❏ Turkey breast, sliced

❏ Low-sodium ham, sliced

❏ Lean roast beef (on occasion), sliced

❏ Lean beef cuts (there's a list of twenty-nine of them on www.beefitswhatsfordinner.com)

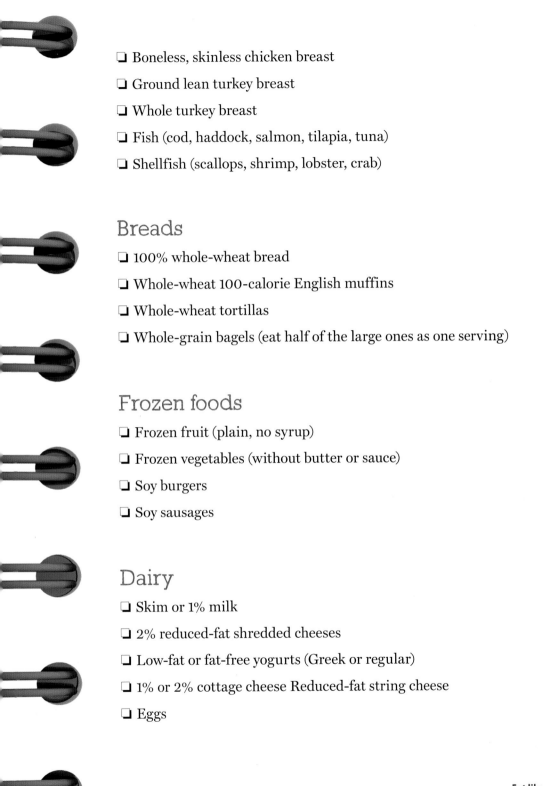

- ❏ Boneless, skinless chicken breast
- ❏ Ground lean turkey breast
- ❏ Whole turkey breast
- ❏ Fish (cod, haddock, salmon, tilapia, tuna)
- ❏ Shellfish (scallops, shrimp, lobster, crab)

Breads

- ❏ 100% whole-wheat bread
- ❏ Whole-wheat 100-calorie English muffins
- ❏ Whole-wheat tortillas
- ❏ Whole-grain bagels (eat half of the large ones as one serving)

Frozen foods

- ❏ Frozen fruit (plain, no syrup)
- ❏ Frozen vegetables (without butter or sauce)
- ❏ Soy burgers
- ❏ Soy sausages

Dairy

- ❏ Skim or 1% milk
- ❏ 2% reduced-fat shredded cheeses
- ❏ Low-fat or fat-free yogurts (Greek or regular)
- ❏ 1% or 2% cottage cheese Reduced-fat string cheese
- ❏ Eggs

The Inner Aisles

- ❏ Dried or canned beans (black, kidney, pinto, black-eyed peas)
- ❏ Lentils
- ❏ Whole-grain cereal (Cheerios, Kashi Heart to Heart, Quaker Oatmeal Squares, Shredded Wheat)
- ❏ Old-fashioned rolled or steel-cut oats
- ❏ Brown rice
- ❏ Whole-grain crackers
- ❏ Whole-grain pasta
- ❏ Almond butter
- ❏ All-natural peanut butter
- ❏ Trail mix
- ❏ Olive oil
- ❏ Canola or vegetable oil
- ❏ Nonstick cooking spray
- ❏ Light mayonnaise
- ❏ Light salad dressings

CHAPTER 6

Eating Out

It's All About Choices

Most nutrition experts say that if you want to lose weight, it's best to eat most of your meals at home, where it's easier to eat right. True, but that advice doesn't always work in the real world. At least, not in my world. My life (and the lives of most kids and families I know) is nuts! My family and I are always on the move, so we eat on the go. So when I started my journey, I knew I had to learn how to make smart choices at our normal restaurant hangouts. I did, and now eating out is almost as easy as eating at home.

Take yesterday, for example. It was a special day—the first day of football practice in full pads—so I had to move. I put a cup of 1% milk and a scoop of protein powder in the blender and added a sliced banana. Thirty seconds later, breakfast! Actually, I made two shakes, one for Mom. Then we headed for the gym so I could get in an early workout.

An hour later, Dad, Kaila, and Zack picked me up. We went to Dick's Sporting Goods to pick up some mouth guards for practice and then argued about where to have lunch. Kaila won: Subway.

I used to eat a whole foot-long loaded with double meat and cheese, chips, a cookie, and a large soda. Not anymore. I ordered a *six-inch* grilled sweet onion chicken sub loaded with veggies on a whole-wheat roll and had the server scoop out the middle of the roll. I washed it down with water and was good to go.

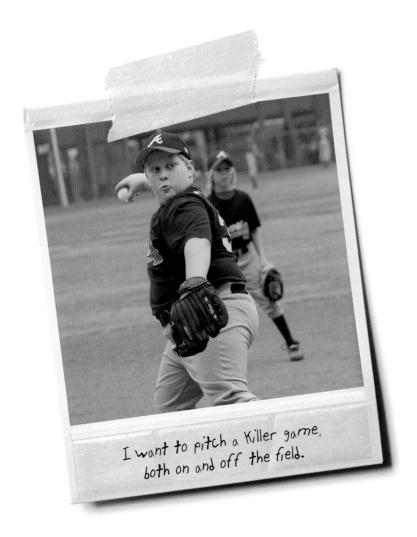

I want to pitch a killer game, both on and off the field.

Then we drove to Dad's office (and mine). By the time Dad finished work and I finished returning Team Tiger emails, it was time for practice, so I ate some rotisserie chicken and hummus—we keep healthy food in the fridge at the office—and drank more water. (A couple of years ago, by this time of day, I would have emptied maybe a couple two-liter bottles of cola.)

After an awesome two-hour workout in near hundred-degree heat, we hit my favorite wing place, Taco Mac, for dinner with some of the team. Instead of the ten wings, soup, cheese dip, Philly cheesesteak, fries, and soda I used to have (boy, when you actually write it out, that's a lot of food), I ordered a grilled chicken breast with buffalo sauce on the side, grilled veggies, and fruit along with a Powerade Zero that tasted like an orange Popsicle. Not long after we got home, I was whooped, so it was off to sleep.

Even if your life is less hectic than this, maybe you can relate. Maybe you're in the school band, on the chess team, or in a bowling league and your team always has dinner before or after practice or the game. Or if your mom or dad works, maybe they bring home takeout a lot because they're too tired or busy to cook. Or maybe they just hate to cook. The point is, people eat out for a lot of reasons, including because it's fun to share a good meal with friends and family.

It's easier than you think to make good choices at a restaurant, the mall, or even the school cafeteria. Team Tiger is about how little changes can add up to big results, and eating out is no exception. Today I go to my favorite hangouts with my team after practice or a game and eat pretty much what they eat. I just customize—you might say "Tigerize"—my order so it's healthier.

I'm not on a diet that I might "break" if I hang with my friends or just be the kid that I am, and you don't have to be either. Just make smart decisions when you eat on the go. You can even treat yourself every now and then as long as you make healthy choices most of the time. Yes, we can—follow me. I'll show you how!

Step 1:
Order things not on the menu.

When my family and I go to restaurants, we're never embarrassed to ask waiters and chefs to make food the way we like it: healthy and tasty. Doing this isn't rude. It's taking control of your health by eating smart. And sometimes, being smart is ordering what's *not* on the menu.

It's funny—no matter what restaurant I go to, I never really read the menu. Too many choices, most of them unhealthy, and sometimes, too much temptation. I already know what foods are healthy—seafood, lean meat, veggies, salads, fruits. So I order those foods, no matter what's on the menu.

Here's a little trick you can use to help you to make better choices:

L Less cheese, more veggies.

E Eat small portions.

A Ask for dressings, sauces, and gravies on the side.

N No fries or fried foods.

It spells out LEAN, which is what you'll be if you use this trick at restaurants!

Say I'm at a burger joint. The menu says I can have a huge cheeseburger with all the trimmings, large fries, and a large drink for one low price. Who cares that you get more food this way? I'd rather spend a little more to eat a lot healthier.

So I pass up the "bargain" and order a regular cheeseburger or grilled chicken sandwich (I eat only half the bun) and a garden salad with light dressing instead of fries.

Or say I'm at a steak house. The menu offers me a combo plate: a steak grilled in butter, a loaded baked potato, soup, and bread and butter. I'll order the steak without the butter and request a double order of vegetables instead of the potato. Also, I don't want the salad bar—instead, I would like a garden salad with light dressing, please, and hold the bacon bits, cheese, and croutons. When you're polite, restaurant staff are usually glad to help you choose healthier options, even if you're ordering something that isn't on the menu. In fact, so many people are trying to lose weight, they're used to special requests!

I just went through this today. We were out running errands and I had just finished my workout and was ready for lunch. We went into a Chinese restaurant we used to go to all the time and now is under new ownership. I didn't feel like plain old steamed chicken and broccoli, so I asked the server if they could stir-fry chicken, shrimp, broccoli, and onion with very little oil and some pepper seasoning, medium spicy.

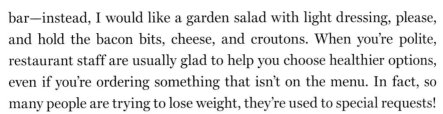

Meet the Team Tiger Expert!

Shane Thompson,
founder, Shane's Rib Shack franchises

I first met Tiger in 2010 when a guy who owned one of my franchises said, "You have to meet this kid." So Tiger, his dad, and I set up a meeting. I was very impressed with Tiger's commitment to fighting obesity. I've fought it almost my whole life, and his passion touched me.

At the Georgia Dome, when I brought out my old suit—the one I wore when I weighed four hundred pounds—I could see the hope in the kids' eyes. These kids don't want to be obese. They are yearning for help and support. It was an honor to be a part of Team Tiger, and I hope to repeat the experience. It's gratifying to see big kids get the help they need from a kid who's been there, and to be a part of that.

> In 2002, Shane Thompson quit his corporate job in medical sales and opened Shane's Rib Shack in McDonough, Georgia. In 2006, he reached his top weight of four hundred pounds, but underwent bariatric surgery in 2007. For the past four years, he has maintained his current weight of about two hundred twenty-five pounds. Now, there are sixty-nine Shane's Rib Shacks nationwide, all offering healthy menu options.

The server didn't get it—he kept showing me stuff on the menu with *sauces*. My dad helped out and nicely asked if the manager could come to our table, so he could explain the dish I wanted. She understood, and I got the healthy, tasty dish I wanted rather than a fatty, unhealthy dish I didn't. So, guys and girls, be nice but be persistent!

One more thing: when you scan a menu, be on the lookout for "bad words." Now, I just said I don't really read menus. But it's always good to know which items to avoid! High-fat, high-calorie foods are described in certain ways, and you have to crack the code. Trust me on this—don't order anything the menu calls crispy, crunchy, battered, fried, au gratin, scalloped, creamy, cheesy, large, grande, supreme, ultimate, sampler, combo, home-style, or country-style. All those words mean one thing: bad news.

Step 2:
Downsize portions.

We've talked about how to practice portion control at home, but you can do it when you eat out too. I know nutrition experts have a lot of drawings and photos and stuff they use to try to help kids (and adults!) visualize portion sizes—that is, how much of any given food you should have on your plate. And I'm going to give you some photos.

That picture (opposite, top)? That used to be my favorite meal when I went to Shane's. You've got your *fried* chicken tenders. A Big Dad barbecue sandwich and fries. A cup of Brunswick stew. Fried okra *and*, for dessert, banana pudding. And not one but four large sodas. If you've ordered a meal that looks like this, don't feel bad. Just look at the next photo (opposite, bottom).

Now that's what I'm talkin' about. You've got your *grilled* tenders, a salad with light ranch dressing, and some fresh green beans, with water to wash it down with. See the difference? I sure do!

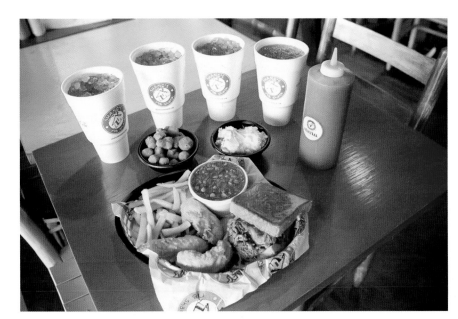

OMG, my stomach hurts just looking at this. No wonder I always felt sick!

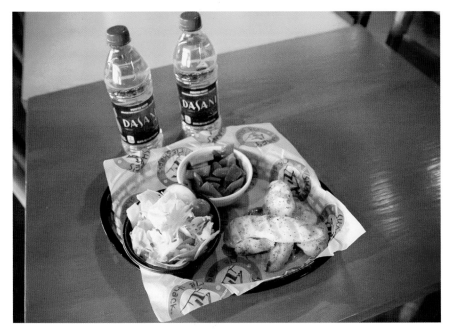

From Supersized to Tigerized!

A Tiger's Tale

Two close friends of ours own restaurants. Charlie owns our favorite barbecue place, a Shane's Rib Shack franchise. Joe owns Taco Mac. After I appeared on Dr. Oz's show, both added healthier choices to their menus. They'd planned to anyway—as dads, they wanted to stay healthy for their families and also believed that offering healthier choices to their customers was the right thing to do—but my determination to get healthy kind of pushed them into action.

It was Charlie who introduced us to Shane, who founded Shane's Rib Shack and agreed to run the Team Tiger station about eating at the Georgia Dome. Shane was perfect for the job because just a few years before, he'd weighed four hundred pounds. He'd had surgery to lose weight, and though he'd lost two hundred pounds by the time of my camp, he was there to show the kids that if they lost weight now, they wouldn't need to do what he'd had to do. I can still see him, putting on the huge suit he'd worn to his daughter's wedding—Shane and I can literally both fit inside the pants now—telling the kids that he was there to help them change now, while they had their whole lives in front of them. He could really relate, and he really cared. He wanted to spare them from the pain and health problems that being heavy had put him through.

Shane also happens to be an awesome cook. That's why I wanted him to run this station. Although one of Team Tiger's first sponsors was a mega-successful organic food chain, I wasn't sure "Eat organic!" was a message that big kids could get excited about. But I was pretty sure they'd listen to a guy who makes the best grilled-chicken tenders I've ever eaten in my life! Shane and Charlie fed almost a thousand kids and parents at the Georgia Dome that day—grilled chicken, chopped chicken barbecue on whole-wheat buns (if they wanted buns), fresh green beans, salad, and small helpings of mac and cheese—and I truly believe that Shane's story helped me change some lives too—parents' as well as kids'.

When it comes to portions, all you really need to know is this: almost everything you *like* to eat—meat, burgers, potatoes, French fries, pie, cake, chips, mac and cheese, whatever—should fit in the palm of your hand. The only exceptions: fruit and veggies. If they're not drenched in cheese, butter, or sauce, you can eat as much of them as you want. And yes, I know that a doughnut or a giant chocolate-chip muffin will fit in your hand, but there are always exceptions to every rule (and this isn't a rule, but a guideline). So use the common sense your mama and daddy gave you to make the healthiest choice you can. I know you got this.

This little guideline really helps when you're eating at a restaurant. No, you shouldn't scoop up your food and put it in your hand—but you can eyeball what's on your plate and push the amount that won't fit into your hand to the side. Or you can ask your mom and dad to help you do this.

If the restaurant you eat at is known for huge portions, ask for a half portion. Some restaurants actually list half portions on their menu (but even if they don't, I ask, and I usually get!). If they don't have half portions, maybe your mom or dad, or another family member, will split it with you. Or you can ask that half of your meal be wrapped to go *before* it's served to you.

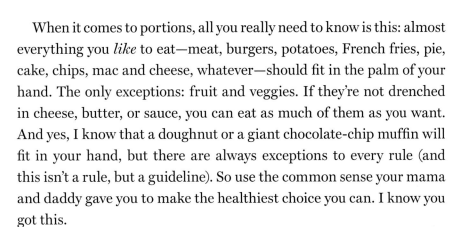

Step 3:
Rack up Tiger points.

Here are some simple ways to make better choices at any restaurant. Any time you eat out, use as many of these suggestions as you can. When we use the term "Tiger points" we aren't asking you to keep track like some of those diet plans—just take notice. When you recap your success for the day, a Tiger point is a pat on the back—like "I get one point for drinking water instead of soda."

Drink two glasses of water with your meal. As soon as you take your seat, drink a glass of water or order a diet drink—diet soda or tea is fine. Have at least one more glass as you're eating. I discovered that water makes food taste a lot better—you are able to taste everything in your food without the weird aftertaste of a sugary drink.

Blow off the bread basket. When you go out to dinner, chances are you'll be brought a basket of bread. Get into a new habit: look at the other tables around you. Do you see a bread basket? If you do, tell your server not to bring one to your table. You've got a whole meal ahead of you—don't fill up on bread!

Sometimes, though, you're eating with people who want the bread. If they do, push the basket their way so it's not in front of you. Or do what I do, start playing drums with it or throw it like a football to your dad so no one wants to eat it after you've had your paws all over it. I promise the waiter won't bring another basket, and when your mom looks horrified, blame it on your pursuit of a healthier lifestyle and some moron named Tiger.

Swap fries for something green. Okay, so vegetables may not be your favorite thing. But you probably like, or at least can deal with, at least one, so order that one. (By the way, the more you eat veggies, the more you end up liking them. These days, I pretty much dig veggies. Try grilled squash and zucchini if it's on the menu, or ask your mom or dad if they'll make it for dinner one night. You slice it up, brush on a little light olive oil or a drop of margarine, sprinkle it with a little lemon pepper, and grill it for a few minutes. It's awesome.)

Most places will let you substitute a salad or a fresh veggie for fries. Sometimes I order *two* green foods—a salad and a vegetable I like. That means I have less room for the stuff I know isn't good for me, like fries, mac and cheese, or potato salad. (If you order two green foods, give yourself a pat on the back and an extra point.)

Pick one: mayo or cheese. When you order a sandwich or burger, decide whether you want cheese or mayo. You'll save a lot of fat and calories if you pick just one. If you choose cheese, stick to one slice. If you choose mayo, ask for it on the side and use a tablespoon or less. But it's not too tough to switch to mustard and lay off the cheese a bit.

Learn to say, "On the side." When it comes to salad dressing, ask for it on the side and you'll use a lot less. Try this trick: dip your fork into your dressing, and then spear the lettuce and veggies. You get all the flavor but less fat and fewer calories. Ask for gravy and sauces on the side too.

Ditch dessert. At my house, dessert is a treat, not an everyday thing. I'm not saying don't ever have dessert; I just make it something I have on special occasions. At a birthday party, have a single slice of cake. And on the last day of school, treat yourself to a small ice cream cone. The operative word is *treat*. The good thing about rethinking dessert is that when you do have it, you'll really enjoy it! At restaurants, if you really want dessert, make it fruit. If they offer a fruit cup on their breakfast menu, and if you ask nicely, I bet they'll be happy to bring you one after dinner! My favorite dessert is a slice of watermelon—you might find that, or some of your favorite fruit, at the salad bar, so ask if you can have a plate of that as your dessert.

Tigerize a Fast-Food Salad

Stopping at a fast-food place for lunch or dinner? Have a burger if you want one, but make it grilled. Chicken salads are an awesome choice too. They fill you up, you get protein in the chicken, you get a serving of green stuff, and they actually taste good!

Here's the thing about salads: they're only as healthy as the stuff that's in them. Here's a major clue: the more green stuff and real veggies you see (cherry tomatoes, broccoli, cucumbers, carrots), the healthier the salad. If you see a lot of ingredients that aren't veggies, chances are it's not as healthy as you think.

Here are some ways to make sure your fast-food grilled-chicken salad is actually a smart choice:

- Make sure the chicken in your salad is grilled, not crispy or fried.

- Be picky about your dressing. This is where an otherwise healthy salad can go all wrong. Use the lowest-fat, lowest-calorie dressing on the menu—either diet or light. Remember, dip your fork into the dressing, then fork up your salad rather than pouring all of the dressing onto your salad.

- A lot of salads at fast-food places come with extras like cheese, bacon bits, and croutons. Instead of getting all three, choose just one. (Pick off the croutons if you have to!)

- If you go to a Mexican fast-food place, stay away from salads served in those crispy bowls that you can eat—I love them, but they really rack up the calories! Instead, order a salad that comes in a bowl you can't eat.

- Here's another good tip for when you order a salad at a Mexican fast-food place: instead of creamy dressings, try your salad "fresco-style." Your salad will be served with a "dressing" that's sort of like fresh salsa. It's really different but really good!

- Instead of ordering fries with your salad, have apple slices or a fruit cup for dessert.

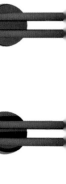

It's Easy to Tigerize When You Go LEAN

Remember, you're not on a diet—you're making better choices. These guidelines can help you do that, and you won't believe how quickly using them becomes a habit.

After you use them a few times, the folks at the restaurant will remember your new "usual order" every time you come in. So just remember LEAN—as in, lean, mean, fighting machine. We are fighting a very personal battle, and we are going to win!

Know Your Restaurants!

You can rack up Tiger points at any restaurant, from your favorite local hangout to a new place you're eyeing on vacation. But it never hurts to be prepared! Here's a cheat sheet that tells you what to order, where.

A burger joint

Because we're always on the go, sometimes there's no alternative but to get off the highway and hit the drive-through. But fast food is more than burgers!

Tiger's healthier choices: I love grilled chicken, so I'll order a grilled-chicken sandwich with mustard instead of mayo. I usually add lettuce and tomato (and a few slices of pickle to add flavor), with fruit for dessert. If I really crave a burger, I'll get one. But not one of those monster burgers with bacon, cheese, and dressing. I order a regular burger with cheese, lettuce, tomato, ketchup, and mustard. Sometimes I eat the bun, sometimes I don't. But if I do, I skip the fries and order a garden salad.

A sub shop

Sub shops like Subway definitely have healthy choices you can sink your teeth into. Order a small (six-inch) sub and fill it with lean meats rather than sausage or meatballs. To round out the meal, you might add a small cup of soup (clear, not creamy) or a small salad with light dressing.

Tiger's healthier choices: Try a six-inch roast beef, chicken teriyaki, or honey mustard chicken sandwich, with no cheese or only one slice. Ask your server to scoop out your whole-wheat or whole-grain roll, request mustard instead of mayo (or light mayo if you hate mustard), and pile on the veggies (lettuce, tomato, and cucumber or banana peppers if you like spicy foods). Veggies add nutrients, crunch, and heft to your sandwich so you'll feel full on less!

A chain restaurant

When you eat at a national chain (like Applebee's, Ruby Tuesday, or Olive Garden), you can feel like it's a celebration—and sometimes it is. These chains sometimes offer a healthier-choice menu, or at least healthy options, but don't be afraid to customize your order!

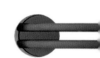

Tiger's healthier choices: Remember the LEAN formula, swap the fatty appetizers for a shrimp cocktail or a cup of clear soup, and you'll do great! The Applebee's menu features several items created in partnership with Weight Watchers and also allows you to order half portions of some platters, which is great. Olive Garden's Garden Fare menu offers some dishes that total fewer than 500 calories. If you get one of these meals, you can also have a salad with light dressing or a cup of minestrone soup.

A barbecue joint

If you're from the South, like I am, you know how important it is to be able to go to your favorite barbecue joint! There are plenty of healthy options to choose from as long as you avoid the fatty sides like mac and cheese or potato salad. (If you just gotta have the mac, split it with a friend or sibling or your mom or dad.)

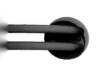

Tiger's healthier choices: Get a grilled chicken salad or grilled chicken tenders seasoned with lemon pepper, rather than smothered in sauce, and a fresh veggie. Or have a barbecue plate with one piece of barbecue chicken, a veggie, and slaw. If you want a barbecue sandwich, get it—just take off the top bun.

A Chinese place

Chinese food is more than egg rolls, fried rice, and sweet-and-sour chicken! Chinese places can do magic things with lean meats, veggies, and a wok—all of them healthy, if you know what to ask for.

Tiger's healthier choices: Clear soup with veggies or lettuce wraps instead of egg rolls are good starters. Then order stir-fried seafood, chicken, bean curd (tofu), or vegetable dishes. My favorite: a stir-fried salt-and-pepper chicken or shrimp with broccoli and asparagus. Rather than the usual side of fried rice, ask for steamed white rice—or brown or purple rice, if the restaurant serves it. (Purple rice—also called "forbidden rice"—is the healthiest of all types of rice. Some Chinese restaurants offer it,

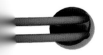

and it's delicious!) Ask your server to have your dish made with less oil too.

An Italian restaurant

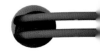

Once you get past the bread or breadsticks, the fatty pasta sauces made with meat or cheese, or the veal or chicken parmesan, then you can get to the healthy stuff. And yes, you can have pasta if you watch your portions and order healthier sauces.

Tiger's healthier choices: Ask your server if you can order pasta in a smaller (lunch) portion, regardless of the time of day. Then top it with a light sauce, like marinara or marsala (wine, mushrooms, beef stock). Seafood is also a great choice when you eat Italian—Italians love their fish.

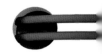

A Japanese restaurant

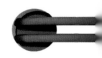

It's amazing how many foods at Japanese restaurants are deep-fried, especially foods with the word *tempura* in the name. Luckily, there are plenty of other foods to choose from.

Tiger's healthier choices: As an appetizer, try a salad or a clear soup, and then ask for broiled, grilled, or steamed items. Broiled fish, grilled chicken, and sushi, sushi, sushi! Because the calories in rice really add up, stick to four to six pieces of sushi. Sometimes you can get sushi made with brown rice, which is healthier than white.

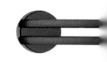

A Mexican place

You'll probably have to order something that's not on the menu at Mexican places—the foods you probably love, like quesadillas, chimichangas, enchiladas, and burritos, aren't the healthiest options. But when you go off menu, you'll do just fine.

Tiger's healthier choices: Tell your server not to bring fried tortilla chips to your table, and ask for raw veggies (carrot sticks, celery, red peppers) that you can dip in your salsa. A cup of black-bean soup is a great appetizer too. For my main meal, I usually order fajitas—shrimp, chicken, or steak grilled with onions, green peppers, lettuce, and diced tomatoes—and tell them to hold the tortillas. (The inside of fajitas is so good, you don't need the outside.) Oh—and hold the sour cream on *everything*. Use spicy salsa instead. If you really love guacamole (like my dad does), have one or two tablespoons and use your veggies for dipping instead of chips.

Give <u>Your</u> Favorite Restaurant a Makeover!

I told you about Charlie and Taco Joe putting healthier choices on their menus. Their places are some of my favorite hangouts, so I'm there a lot—and I always see people ordering the healthier stuff along with the not-so-healthy stuff. The fact that they have a choice makes me feel really good.

But did I tell you I forced my own grandma to offer healthier items on her menus?

Here's the story: Grandma runs the concession stands at five of the Little League parks around Atlanta, and I occasionally work at the stand for her, selling hot dogs and ice cream bars and all the stuff you eat at Little League games. Right after I was on Dr. Oz's show, Grandma called and asked me to work at one of her stands.

"Not until you put healthier choices on your menu," I said. (I still can't believe I told my own grandma no.)

"Okay," Grandma said, "but I don't know if people will buy them. They want hog dogs and ice cream. But I love you, and I'll give it a shot."

"They will. I'll prove it to you," I said. "I know what kids like me will eat if you give them a chance—and, by the way, Grandma—it's not a bad idea for you either." (Did I mention she has amazingly good accuracy when she swings her cane at me?) So that day, before I went to the stand to work, Dad and I went to the supermarket and bought chicken breasts, whole-wheat buns, apples, and carrots. We lugged it all over to the concession stand, put the chicken on the grill, and started slicing and wrapping the carrots and apples. Then I taped a sign on the concession-stand window that listed the healthier options.

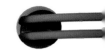

I sat outside, grilling the chicken, while people walked by and asked if we were selling it or if it was just for me. "No, I'm actually cooking this for all of you," I said.

I'll put it this way: we sold every bit of our healthier menu within the first hour!

Now all the stands that offer the Team Tiger healthier choice menu are sponsored by Whole Foods Market, and these healthier options— including low-fat milk, Nutri-Grain and fiber bars, fresh fruit, turkey

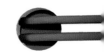

From: **Zack**
Subject: **Team Tiger Member**

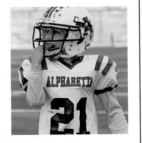

Hi, I'm Zack. Tiger's little brother. Even though I'm only eight years old, I've learned a lot in the last two years while Tiger has been on his journey. I learned that exercise is not work—it's fun—and I found some things that I love and do every day. Biking, football, basketball, and hiking are some of my favorite activities! I just got a new puppy, and I've been walking him every day. I know exercise is important but eating right is also part of being healthy. At school I see a lot of people who need Tiger's help, and I take them through the first steps. Tiger has taught me a lot, and without him I would not be who I am today.

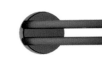

dogs, and Powerade Zero—have become over 60 percent of the total food sales. If you give kids better options, they'll make better choices. It's not just what I think. It's what I've seen!

Now that you've started your own journey, look around you. Is there a local restaurant you know of that might offer healthier choices? Could they offer steamed veggies along with their fries and onion rings, or grilled chicken sandwiches along with their burgers?

Maybe you could ask the owners about putting a few healthy options on their menus. It can't hurt to ask. Just make sure you have a few suggestions. If you succeed, you've helped people you don't even know make better choices, and you can feel good about that.

Hangin' at the Mall: Healthy Options at the Food Court

The last time I ate at the mall, I had a plate of teriyaki shrimp and vegetables with sauce on the side from that Japanese place that's at every mall in the world. Did I feel deprived? No way. My choice was tastier and healthier than the pizza, burgers, and fried chicken sandwiches most of my friends ordered. (I'm happy to say that a couple of them went with my choice.)

Now, I could have ordered an even *healthier* dish—steamed chicken and broccoli at the Chinese place—but I wasn't in the mood for it. So my choice wasn't perfect. But it was way healthier than a lot of other options, and I can live with that.

Maybe you're thinking the food court at your mall doesn't offer any healthy foods. Well, the next time you're hanging at the mall with your friends and they want to eat, chill. I'll bet you can find these:

- Pizza place: a single slice of thin-crust veggie pizza

- Chinese place: stir-fried chicken, shrimp, or beef with veggies, hold the egg roll and fried rice

- Salad place: a salad with some type of lean protein—grilled chicken or turkey—and a cup of clear soup

- Burger joint: a small hamburger with a side salad or a grilled chicken breast sandwich, hold the special sauce, and skip the fries

- Diner: a sandwich on whole-grain bread, skip the fries and chips (If the sandwiches at the place are as thick as one of your library books, ask them to use half the meat and cheese.)

- Ice cream place: a sugar-free frozen yogurt cone

I feel great about being able to choose healthy foods among so many unhealthy options (including those soft pretzels that are as big as your head!). Being able to pick out the few healthy choices among the many unhealthy ones is a skill *you* can be proud to show off too.

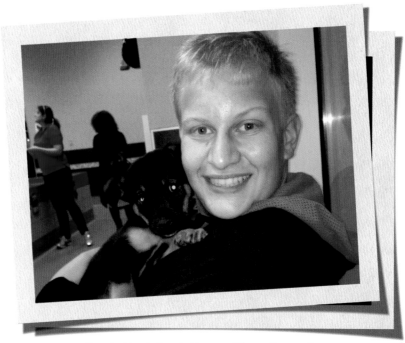

Meet the latest Team Tiger Expert: an expert in cuddling!

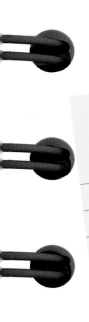

Chalk Talk with My Dad:
How Parents Can Help

I love dining out, and going to restaurants we enjoy is a bonding experience for Tiger and me. I ate lunch with my dad almost every weekday for fifteen years when we worked together. We didn't talk much, but it was *our* way of bonding.

But when Tiger started on his journey, I realized that, like him, I'd have to change the way I thought about dining out—and change what I ordered too. Now, we've learned how to enjoy the experience and time together in a healthier way.

One of the biggest lessons Marsha and I learned was that Tiger really *wanted* to make better choices—he just needed support. If you make good choices, so will your children. If you order less, your children will too. And you can help them order less in small ways that don't shame them. For example, you might quietly take the waiter aside and cancel that appetizer, then replace the time you'd spend eating those mozzarella sticks or chicken wings with just talking—about school, what their day was like, or what books they're reading. Chances are, your children won't even miss the appetizer.

Then later, in private, congratulate them on choosing such healthy meals and use that positive restaurant outing to build on. You can also help your children scan the menu and pick out healthier choices. ("Remember what you ordered when we went to the pizza place? I see they have that here. Want to try that, or I see that there's a steak salad on the menu . . . want to split it with me?")

Above all, be a parent; learn to say no. You'll be glad you did. Tiger didn't need me to be his friend; he needed his father to say no in a supportive way. I often cast him as the hero, as in, "Let's not get that appetizer, 'cause you know I'll eat it all. I need you to help me do the better-choices thing you're doing." ➜

I also find positives to help Tiger build on, like reminding him how well he did the last time he was at a restaurant or how hard he worked that day. ("You just had a great workout, so let's not waste it on these chips. Hey, guys, who wants to take the dogs for a walk when we get home? I need to work off dinner.")

Before we started this journey, I guess I couldn't see all the food Tiger was putting away while my head was in the sand. Now, my head is firmly above ground, and I'm there to support my son, my other kids, and all their friends in making healthy choices—in a gentle but firm and supportive way.

I woke up this morning and checked the obituaries. My name wasn't in them, so it must not be too late to turn things around.

PART 3

Follow Me Into . . . An Active Life

Yes, this is the exercise part of the book. But don't stop reading! Team Tiger is not about perfection. It's about progress and giving it your best effort (heart). I promise I know how you feel about physical activity—I've spent most of my life feeling that way.

I used to get so tired—not just from trying to keep up with the other kids but also from the snickers and comments I got. One day on the playground, right before I started my journey, my friends and I walked by one of the biggest bullies in my school and his followers. "His name may be Tiger, but he looks like an elephant!" he sneered.

One of the biggest changes I made in my journey was that I committed to do something active every single day. I knew there had to be a way that a big kid like me could tackle exercise. As I found out, there was. The workouts in this section are the same drills and exercises that I did from day one of my journey and that are now included at the Team Tiger camps.

The key to my success—and yours too—is to work at a pace that challenges you and just you. You won't be breaking any records for a while, but that doesn't matter. This is your program, based on your definition of success, whether you're a boy or a girl. The activities you'll be doing are pretty much the same ones we offered at our first camp at the Georgia Dome.

My goal each day is to do a little bit better than the day before, no matter how small the increase. Try it. That one extra sit-up will become three, then five, then who knows? That extra thirty-second effort becomes a minute more, then five minutes more, and then . . . well, you get the idea. My point is, those extra sit-ups and seconds add up.

The four activity stations in this section focus on four different types of activities: agility, quickness, strength, and flexibility. In each station, you'll move from drill to drill fairly quickly. Believe me, they'll keep you moving. But you'll be having so much fun that you probably won't even notice!

Do all four activity stations two to three times a week. Do all of the flexibility exercises at every workout, and do them last, when your muscles are good and warmed up.

After you do the agility station, you're ready to tackle the other three stations. To start out, choose one or two exercises from each station and do ten of each. (Doing one exercise, one time, is called a repetition—or a rep, for short.) Once you've been doing the stations for a month, choose three or four exercises from each station and do ten reps. After three months, do all five exercises from each station and perform ten reps each.

Are you a little nervous about tackling this exercise stuff? Don't be. There's no pressure, especially from me. Remember, this is supposed to be fun! And you don't have to compare how well you do to how well anyone else does. You're challenging yourself—to be fitter, to be healthier, to find out how cool it is to get stronger, quicker, and more confident in yourself and your abilities.

So let's get started!

CHAPTER 7

Agility
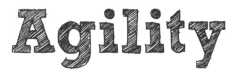

You Zig, I'll Zag

I look up to all good people, but I especially admire the ability of good athletes—not just football players but also basketball players, hockey players, and even golfers. No matter what their game is, they're all light on their feet. In other words, they have *agility*—the ability to change direction while in motion, without slowing down.

When I was heavy, agile I was not. I always had the big-kid shuffle—my feet barely left the ground, partly because I had so little energy and partly because I was carrying too much weight. I knew this foot-dragging was slowing me down, on and off the field. So when Coach Z and I started working together, my agility was one of the first things I asked him to help me improve.

Even if you don't play sports, I want you to know that agility is also a great quality to have at home where, if you're like me, you have a big brother with a mean headlock, a little brother that's the perfect height for permanent damage, a sister with a wicked backhand, a bird that can bite your fingers off, a cat with sharp claws, or a German shepherd puppy nipping and teething on *everything*. (We won't even talk about my miniature pinscher, Scout, and his love of my leg!)

My point: I use agility for family survival too, and so can you. Even though I'll probably always be the big target, I don't have to be the easy target!

The agility drills in this chapter will make you hard to catch— whether you're playing sports, a pickup game of ball or tag with your friends, or eluding aforementioned family members, friends, and pets who are out to get you. The drills are a fun way to get your body moving. You get to challenge yourself, and it won't be long before you notice that your body is reacting more quickly. Work at your own pace, but try to do each drill ten times, resting in between drills as needed.

One more thing: most of these drills are done with cones, which you can buy at most sporting-goods stores or online, but you can use pretty much anything in place of cones, even throw pillows from your couch. You can also use cups, socks, tape, chalk, or spray paint to mark out the places where the cones would go.

The Tale of Tiger Tail

Tiger Tail goes back to my first year of playing football. I was seven, playing with older kids because of my size, and my dad was my coach. Because he worried about how I would feel about not being able to keep up with the other kids during conditioning drills, our team didn't do them much. Instead, we focused on football skills. As a result, the team wasn't as well conditioned as it should have been. Although we had a great season, fatigue definitely affected our performance.

As the season went on, my dad realized that he was not being fair to the team (or to me) by conditioning the other players down to me rather than me up to them. So at the start of our next season, at our first team meeting, he talked to the parents about us kids all learning from everything we do and about how the parents should never stop trying to be better parents and coaches for their kids.

Then I met Coach Z, who worked at my health club. We clicked, and I started working out with him as much as I could.

The next year, when football started again, Dad asked Coach Z to set up a conditioning station for our team. Instead of just running sprints at the end of practice like every other team, Coach Z had us do over an hour of conditioning drills, along with other activities that improved our skills—including our footwork and agility.

One of the things Dad wanted the team to work on was footwork and keeping our heads moving so we'd be better able to follow the play at all times. So Coach Z and I came up with Tiger Tail, a combination of conditioning, skill, and fun. Tiger Tail was one of our team's favorite activities.

I liked it too. In fact, for one of the first times in my life, I was good at an exercise. I learned you don't have to be the fastest to be the quickest. It was cool to know that I could get either in or out of someone's way easily enough to make quickness a very effective weapon. It also taught me how to use my body to block someone from getting to my tail. (At times, size can be an advantage!) This was really cool and fun to me, and I was good at it, so I started to gain confidence in football—and in life.

One other thing: for the first time in my life, I started thinking with that "glass half full" mentality. I learned that I was athletic, quick, and smart enough to use my size as a positive force. I saw that I could build on these positives to go forward rather than dwelling on the negatives and allowing them to hold me back.

I got all this from a really simple activity that is a lot of fun!

Tiger Tail

This is one of my favorite drills. You'll need at least one other person to do this activity with you, so get your friends or family to join in—the more people, the more fun! You'll also need a "tail" for each player—a bandana, a sock, or even a piece of duct tape works great. Play it each night with your family to see who gets to pick your healthy dinner!

1. Set up 4 cones so they form the outside of a large imaginary rectangle, as opposite. Make sure your rectangle is large enough to run around in—the bigger, the better!

2. Get all the players to form a circle inside the rectangle. The size of the circle depends on the number of people playing, but it should be big enough to have everybody a few feet apart.

3. Have everyone tuck their "tail" into the back of their pants.

4. The goal is to grab everyone else's tail out without them getting yours, so here we go! Staying inside the cones, try to grab the other players' tails. Stay light on your feet and keep moving! If your tail gets pulled, pick it up and go outside the circle to cheer on your friends and wait for this round to finish. The round ends when only one person has a tail still tucked in. That person wins—but remember, everyone who keeps moving gets Tiger points!

5. Play a few rounds, and try to have each round last 5–10 minutes, or until you've captured all but one tail. You'll get a good cardio workout without even realizing it!

Coach Z's Top Tip

When you play Tiger Tail, always shuffle your feet (never cross them), and never stop moving. And as we say in football, "Keep your head on a swivel," which means to keep your eyes on everybody all the time. Last, but not least, like everything else we do, find a positive and build from it. Whether you have good vision, quick feet, or solid logic, you've got a skill that can help in this game.

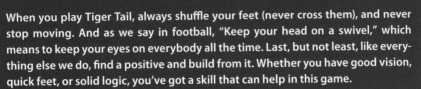
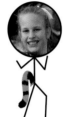
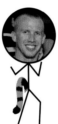
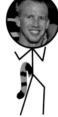

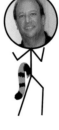
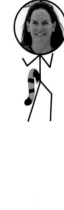
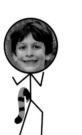
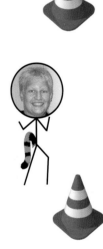

Look how well this drill works! See how skinny we are now!

The T-Drill

This activity develops your footwork and keeps you moving too. You'll be zigzagging in several different directions during this drill, so you might want to "rehearse" it a few times to get the hang of it.

Set up your cones in the shape of the letter *T*. Make sure that the bottom cone (the end of the *T*) is ten yards (about ten big steps) from the top middle cone, and that the cones that form the top of the *T* are five yards (or five big steps) apart.

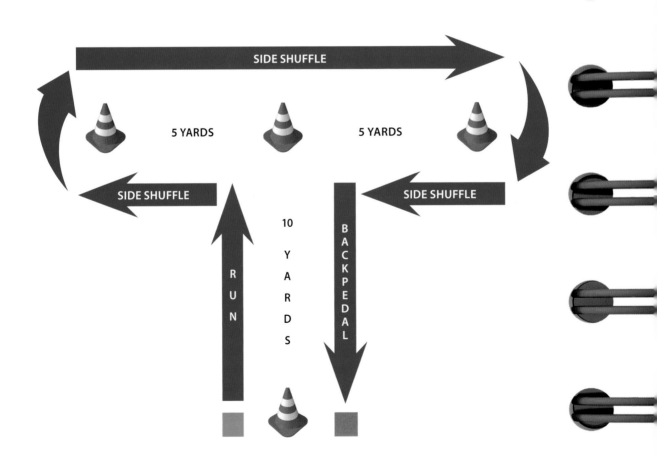

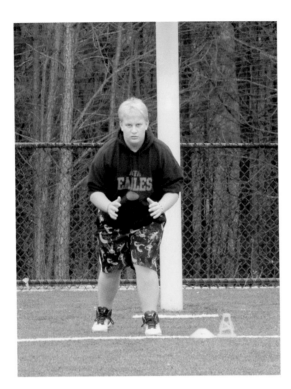

1. Stand at the bottom of the *T*, put one foot in front of another shoulder-width apart (we call this a "plant foot rear" and a "pressure foot front") with your knees slightly bent and your hands and arms balanced in front of you. Now you're in a good athletic stance.

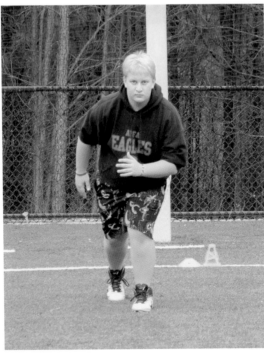

2. Run forward to the top middle cone. Go as fast as you can! It's not a race, but push yourself as best you can—you can do this!

3. From the top middle cone, side shuffle to the left of the *T*. To side shuffle to the left, first step out with your left foot.

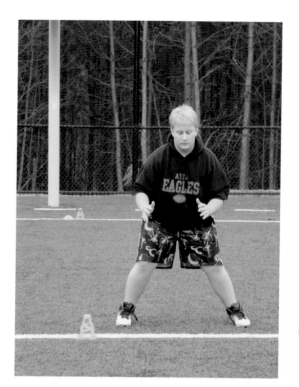

4. Then shuffle your right foot toward your left foot. Make sure not to cross your feet or let your heels touch. This completes a shuffle step. Do it slowly a couple of times until you get used to it.

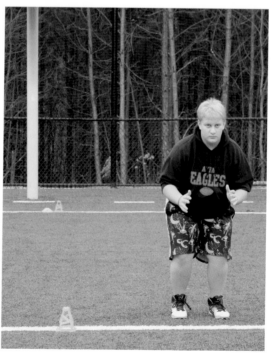

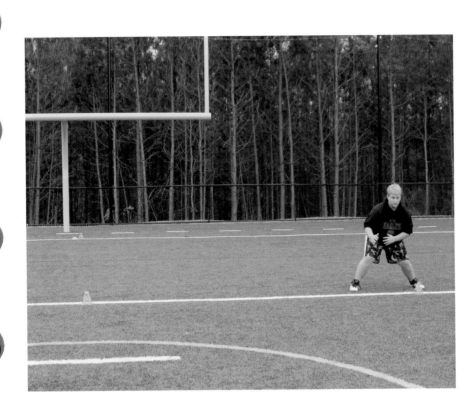

5. When you reach the far left cone, shuffle all the way back to the far right cone, and then back to the middle cone. From the top middle cone, backpedal to the bottom of the *T*. Basically, backpedaling is running backward. When you backpedal, keep your shoulders over your knees so you are leaning forward. (If you stand straight and try to backpedal, you will fall backward—I know this for a fact). Again, do this a few times slowly and then gradually speed up. If you do fall, get up quickly and keep going. Remember, nothing can keep you down anymore—you are your only obstacle. Complete 10 reps.

Cuts

In this drill, you'll work on your ability to change directions, moving left and right. Do the drill at a slower pace the first week or two until you strengthen your knees and ankles. Expect to be a little sore at first, but don't let that stop you. You'll be amazed at how quickly you'll be able to do it.

1. Set up 6 cones about 5 feet apart in a zigzag formation.

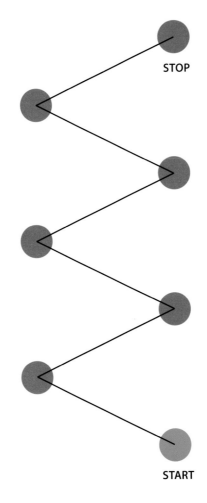

STOP

START

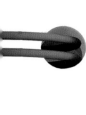

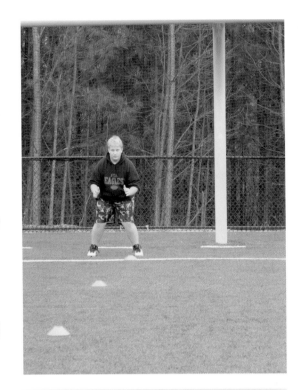

2. Stand with the back cone just in front of your left foot, with your knees slightly bent, shoulder-width apart, and your arms and hands in front of your body. Place your right foot outside of the cone.

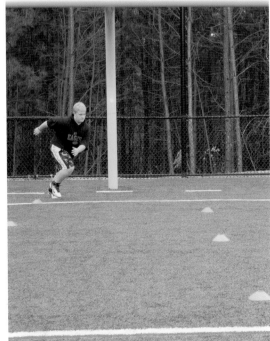

3. Starting with your right foot, step toward the cone on your left. Your right foot should be crossing your body so your body is in position to start sprinting in the direction of the next cone.

4. Run to the first cone.

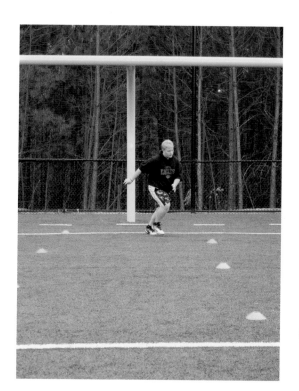

5. Once you reach the cone, plant your outside foot firmly onto the ground and drive back toward the other side until you reach the next cone.

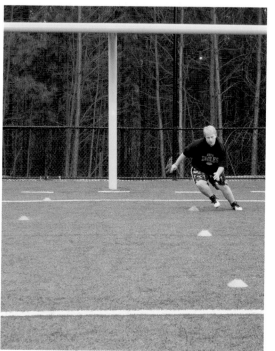

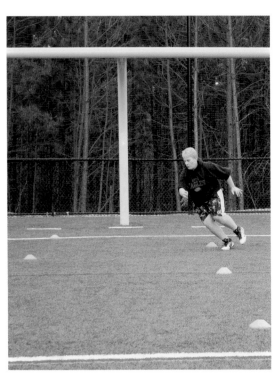

6. Shift your momentum going the other way and sprint to the next cone.

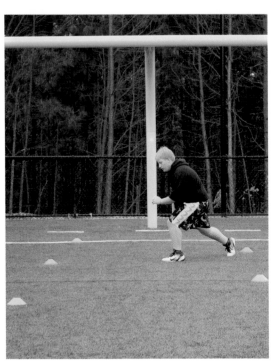

7. When you get to the last cone, run as fast as you can (sprint) a few yards straight ahead. If you are working with a partner, have him or her toss you a ball or something—this will remind you to keep alert and keep your head up. If you're working by yourself, just sprint and smile—you are on your way! Complete 10 reps.

Mark's Story

In 2010, a few weeks before our camp at the Georgia Dome, a reporter at a local TV station interviewed Marcus and me about the event. At the end of the interview, she made her viewers an offer: the first twenty-five people to email the station or post on my Facebook page about why they or their kids wanted to start their own journeys to a healthier, more active lifestyle would get a spot at the camp.

By the time Marcus and I left the studio, my phone was vibrating nonstop—the station was already receiving emails. By the time Dad and I reached our car in the station's lot, all twenty-five spots had been claimed. Although each story was amazing, one will always stick with me.

The mom of a young man who lived in northern Florida emailed me about her son, then twelve years old (just about my age at the time). Six weeks earlier, he had tried to take his own life. I could feel his mother's pain in every word. I thought I knew what was coming next, and I was right.

Mark didn't feel that anyone could understand the pain of being the big kid your entire life. He was flunking out of school and had no friends. Sometimes he didn't go to class. If he did, he found excuses not to participate, or he fought with other boys. He simply couldn't find a reason to go on for another day, and he tried to commit suicide.

Thank God he didn't succeed. During his recovery, his mother wrote, he saw an interview with me (a rerun, no less!) on CNN. When I mentioned the upcoming camp at the dome, his mom said, he smiled for the first time in a long time. She promised she would get him one of the spots at the camp—and with her email, she did.

The day of the camp, before kids began the stations, I saw a young man surrounded by adults walking toward me. I kind of nudged my dad. "We are about to meet Mark," I said. I just knew it was him.

We walked toward them. He'd brought his mother, a teacher, and the principal of his school. I walked up and gave him a "man hug"—shoulder to shoulder—and told him how proud I was of him coming to the camp. I reassured him that better things were to come. Mark was smiling, but his eyes looked determined. In fact, after just about a minute of conversation, he said, "It's time to get to work!" I laughed, nodded, and led him to his group.

During the lunch break, Dad had a chance to talk to Mark's principal and teacher. Three weeks ago, they said, he'd found out he was coming to the camp. Since then, he'd been an entirely different kid. His sense of humor returned, he was participating in class and making friends, and his grades had risen dramatically. Most impressively, he'd begun walking every day with a new group of friends—some of them big like Mark, some not—who responded to his new, positive outlook.

At the end of the camp, I looked for Mark—I wanted to see if he'd enjoyed his day. I could tell from the look in his eye that he would never again feel alone or desperate. He called me about a month after the camp to tell me that he had lost over thirty pounds and had just signed up to play football for the first time. I haven't heard from him in a while, but in a few more years I'll start looking for him in the NFL!

Clockwork Drill

You can have fun with this next drill by having a friend or family member help.

Set up six cones as you see in the diagram—notice that they're numbered in clockwise direction. Place the cones about one yard apart from each other. (There should be seven yards between the top cone and the base cone.)

Have the person working with you stand aside. His or her job is to shout out the numbers of the cones. (You could shout out the numbers yourself, but the neighbors might think you're a little weird. Having a friend or family member yell out the numbers is really just to add to the fun for you!) Whatever number he or she shouts out, run to that cone, touch it, and return to base. That's one rep. Repeat until you have done ten reps.

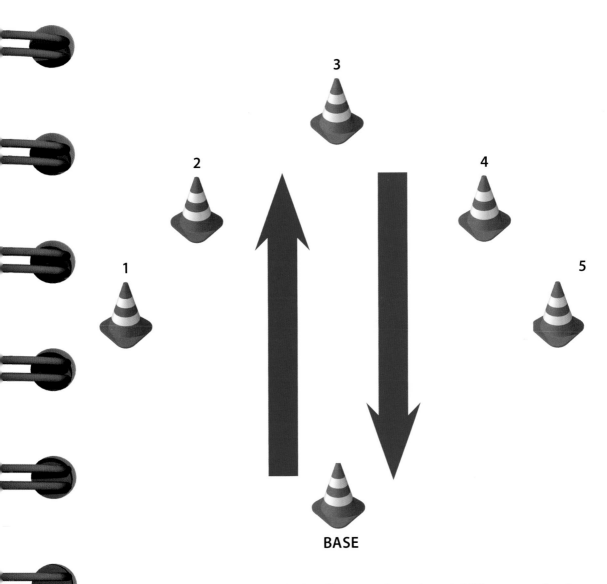

3

2

4

1

5

BASE

Starting at the base cone, have somebody yell out a number, 1 through 5. Whatever number they say, run to that cone, touch it, and return to base. Keep doing this until you reach 10 reps.

In-Out Ladder Drill

There are so many drills you can do with an agility ladder! This drill may sound trickier than it is, but hang in there—it's one of my favorites. You can get good at it quickly, and it keeps your heart rate up, especially if you go straight from the ladder to another activity.

You can buy an agility ladder at a sporting-goods store, or you can make your own—just draw a "ladder," ten 18" x 18" boxes—with chalk or tape on the ground.

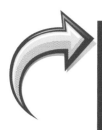

> **Coach Z's Top Tips**
>
> • Once you get pretty good at this drill, get your friends and family to try it. They will think it looks easy until they try it, and then they will be amazed at what you can do. Then, game on—they will want to do it with you. (You got them moving too. Great job!)
>
> • While you're learning these drills, go slowly and focus on doing them right. Once you have the pattern down, then work on getting quicker.
>
> • As you do these drills, keep your head up. It makes the drill more challenging.

1. Stand tall, your arms at your sides, with both feet inside the first square.

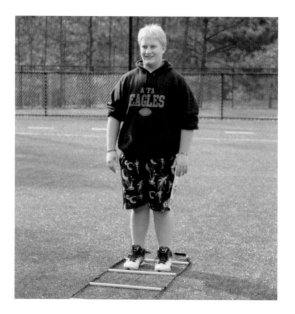

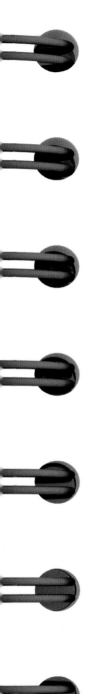

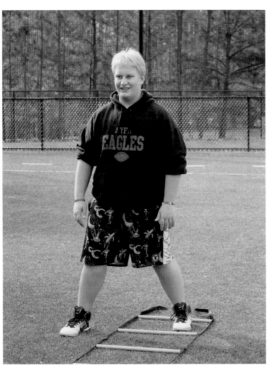

2. With your right foot, quickly high-step outside of the square to the outside of the box in front of you. Keep your back straight and your knees slightly bent.

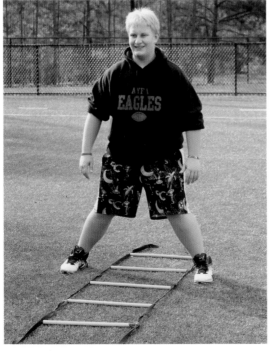

3. Repeat with your left foot. (You don't have to smile, but I always have fun with the ladder drills!)

4. High-step your right foot inside the second box. (Sound familiar? "You put your right foot in and you shake it all about . . ." Just think of what you're doing as an advanced version of the hokey pokey.)

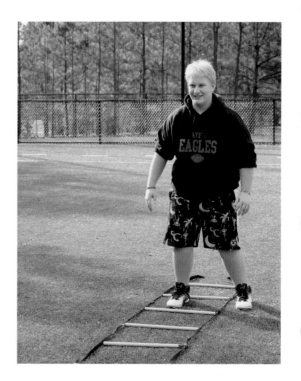

5. High-step your left foot into the box so that both feet are now inside the box. Continue up the ladder until you exit out the other end. When you do, you've completed a rep. Repeat, starting with the left foot first. Complete 10 reps.

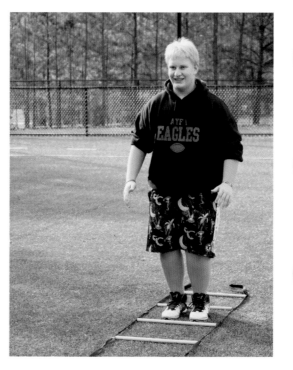

Cardio for a Cause

"Normal" cardio exercise, like walking on a treadmill or pedaling a stationary bike, isn't fun enough for me, so it isn't my favorite way to exercise. But I realize that cardio is a must if you want to lose weight and be healthy. But, being me, I had to find a way to make it fun so I could enjoy making it a bigger part of my life— and I did.

Before I started on my journey, I had never much been into running ('cause I could hardly run at all), so I never would have even considered a 5K—that's a race that's 3.1 miles long. But once I did start running, my mom decided I would be her new running partner. So she signed us up for the Big Peach 5K Run/Walk in Atlanta.

I'd started my journey five months before and had lost about forty pounds. Still, before the race, I had to run from the bathroom to the start line because I got sick—I was freaking out! My mom and Coach Z told me to just do my best, jog as much as I could, and then walk a little until I was ready to jog some more. I finished my first ever 5K in about an hour and was surprised to realize that I felt amazing, both mentally and physically. Well after that, I started trying to match up races (more like fun walk/runs) with charitable causes that I really believed in and wanted to support.

One of my next events was the SOS (Save Our Skin) 5K, a walk/run for skin cancer awareness. I registered in honor of my friend's dad, who had passed away from the disease. So I, together with my friend and his mom, put a Team Tiger group of thirty-five people together. We wore Team Tiger shirts with his dad's picture on them, and we got the award for the largest group participating. I found it so cool having all these friends and parents doing this together that I didn't even realize I had cut my time down to forty-four minutes—a pretty good improvement!

If a kid like me, who once couldn't even jog, can find a way not just to run but to make it fun, I'll bet you can too. How cool would it be, as you're changing yourself for the better—getting fitter, healthier, and more confident in yourself—to support a cause that makes the world a better place too? Plus, you get a new T-shirt! You can find 1K and 5K fun runs for causes you believe in on the Internet—just Google "fun run" and your zip code. Then sign up and do them at your own pace. Hey, help me organize a Team Tiger event like that in your city, and we'll do it together.

CHAPTER 8

Quickness

Catch Me If You Can!

I think almost everyone I know has seen the movie *Dodgeball*. And I know everybody I saw it with cheered for the underdogs. What was the key to the success for the Average Joes? You got it—quickness! Remember Patches O'Houlihan's famous quote: "If you can dodge a wrench, you can dodge a ball!"

None of the quickness drills you'll do involve wrenches. But they will make you faster and more coordinated, improving your ability to do just about anything. I remember a game we used to play at my school, Wall Ball. Basically, you and another kid, or a group of kids, stand facing a wall and someone throws the ball against the wall from wherever he or she is standing. The distance between you and the person throwing the ball varies with every throw, which changes your reaction time. That's part of the challenge—and the fun! If you catch the ball, then you throw it against the wall. If the ball hits you and you don't catch it, you have to run and touch the wall before the other player can throw the ball to the wall. If the ball hits the wall before you do, you're out.

You can see that if you're playing Wall Ball, being big and slow isn't your ideal combination. So at the start of my journey, one of the first things I wanted to work on was quickness. One reason was to dominate at Wall Ball. The other reason, as you probably can guess, was to play better football.

Because I was always the biggest kid on the field, the opposing coaches eventually gave up on trying to put their biggest kid on me. And to be painfully honest, it wasn't that I was that good or strong, I was just that big and immovable.

So their next plan was to get someone small and fast across from me. The other coaches figured they could count on me being pretty slow. But I was doing the drills you'll do in this section, so I had gotten faster, and their plan didn't work so well.

I remember this one game in particular. The opposing coach took out his biggest kid and put a quick, athletic kid in. When the ball was snapped, this kid shot low and quick, trying to get by my right side. He didn't count on me being lower and quicker. I beat him to the spot and hit him so hard that I drove him into the three linemen next to him—they looked like a line of dominoes toppling.

After that game, the coaches of all the other teams realized that they could no longer count on my being slow. Thanks to this station, I

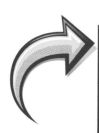

Coach Z's Top Tips

- Quickness drills shouldn't be forced—the goal is to do them right, not to do them fast—at least at first. Keep at it, and you'll soon get faster and faster.

- To make these drills more of a challenge, keep your head up while you do them.

- As you do these drills, think to yourself, "Quick feet, quick feet, quick feet!" That little chant in your head will push your feet to be quicker—for real!

became one of the quickest kids on my team. I also love Wall Ball, and now my brothers and sister aren't so quick to think they can get away with that quick little slap or punch and run!

Even my dog Scout knows I can catch him now. Whenever he gets loose and sees me running after him, he stops and rolls over. (My next book may have to be Team Scout! My dog looks like an oil can with legs. I take his weight as a personal challenge because I think that if your dog is too big, then you aren't getting enough exercise.) Your pet can be your best exercise buddy if you let him. Since the last time Scout got loose, he has done three 5Ks with me.

These drills don't look like much on paper—they're short, and it looks like there's not much to them. But they're surprisingly challenging, and if they're good enough for the NFL, imagine what they'll do for you! When I first started doing these drills, I was lucky if I could jump over my latest copy of *Sports Illustrated*. I started out at my own level, as you should, and just kept trying. Believe me, each time you do them, it will get easier and your speed and clearance will get better.

You can do these drills virtually anywhere—in your driveway, on the sidewalk in front of your house, or in an empty parking lot. Use tape or chalk to draw a line about three feet long. Wear well-cushioned sneakers to do these drills—they'll help protect your knees, joints, and ankles.

Select three of the drills below and do them twice for thirty seconds at a time. An easy way to check your progress is to count how many hops you can do in thirty seconds. Then, two weeks later, see how many you can do in that same period of time. Focus, keep your balance, and be as quick and light on your feet as you can. As you get faster, choose new drills and increase your interval to forty-five or sixty seconds. Really have fun with these drills. You will be surprised by how much these activities come into play in your everyday life.

Now, are you ready? Come on, y'all! Let's do this!

Double Leg Forward and Backward Line Hops

As you start to get good at these drills, you want to hop a little bit higher, farther, and faster, and increase both your jumps per minute and how long you do them (your endurance).

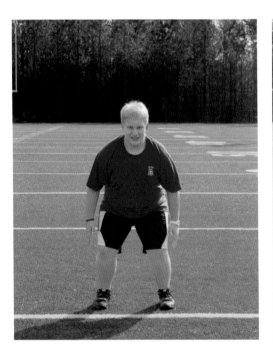

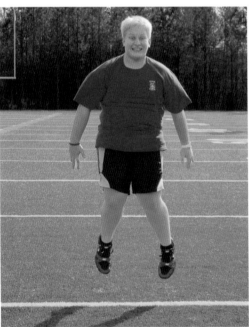

1. Draw or tape a 3-foot line on the floor. Put your hands by your sides, feet shoulder-width apart, toes toward the line, knees bent. You're ready for takeoff!

2. Leap, propelling yourself forward over the line.

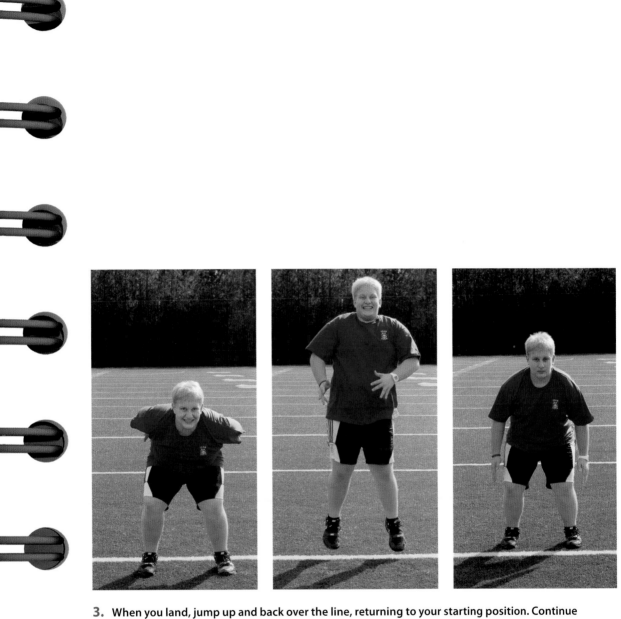

3. When you land, jump up and back over the line, returning to your starting position. Continue quickly jumping forward and then backward over the line for thirty seconds (one rep). Do 10 reps of these.

Double Leg Side-to-Side Line Hops

If you want to make this drill a little more interesting, hop over items that are hurdles in your weight loss journey. During this drill, I sometimes hop over a box of Girl Scout Cookies (I still love Thin Mints) or a six-pack of soda. They're obstacles, but now they won't hold you back! (Just be careful!)

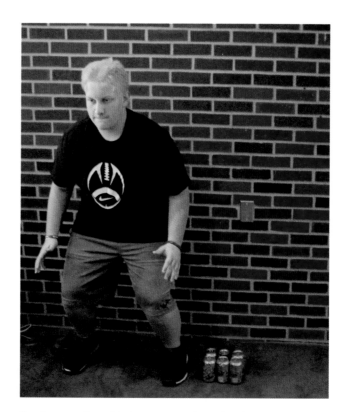

1. Assume the athletic stance to the right of your challenge (in this case, a six-pack of soda), with your feet shoulder-width apart and your knees slightly bent. Keep your arms at your sides and away from your body.

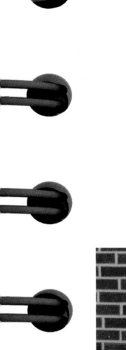

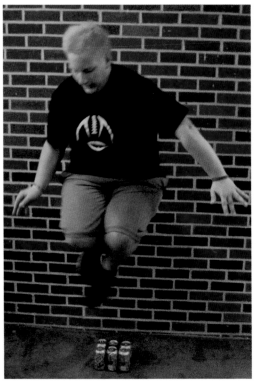

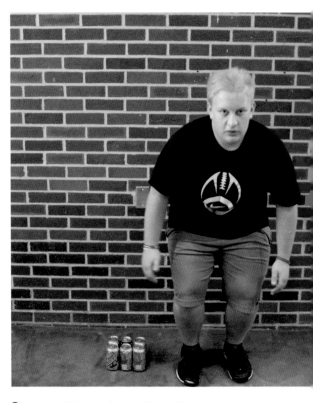

2. Using pressure off your outside foot, jump sideways up and over the challenge, landing on the other side. Jump high, so you'll clear the obstacle with both feet!

3. Land with your knees slightly bent to take the impact off your joints. Regain your balance and then jump back in the other direction. Repeat 10 times.

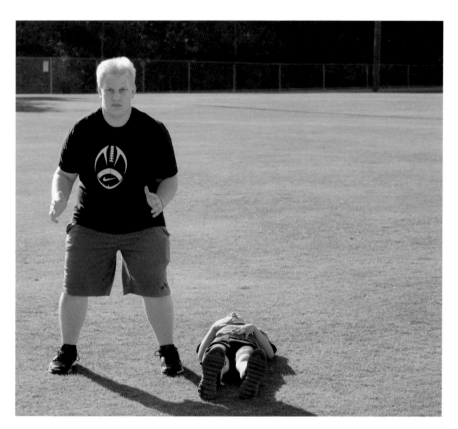

4. Get into an athletic stance to the right of your challenge (in this case, my little brother, Zack) with your feet shoulder-width apart and your knees slightly bent. Keep your arms at your sides and away from your body.

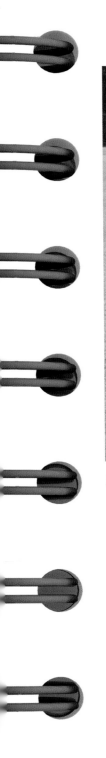

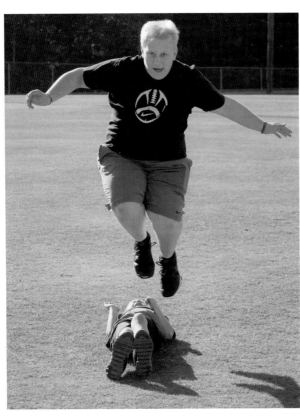 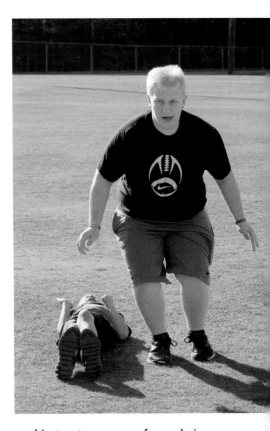

5. Using pressure off your outside foot, jump up and over your object, pet, or person of your choice (I recommend a turtle that won't move out of the way very quickly), landing on the other side. Remember to jump high!

Muhammad Ali Line Shuffle

Float like a butterfly, sting like a bee. Time to do these drills with me!

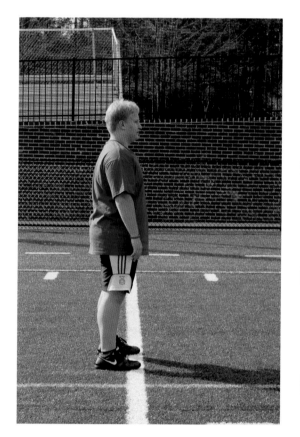

1. **Stand tall with your feet shoulder-width apart.**

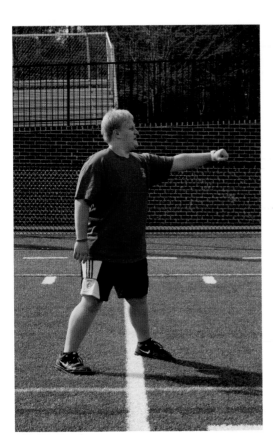

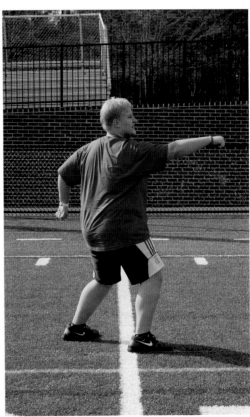

2. Step forward with your left foot and raise your arms at chest level, curling your hands into loose fists. With knees slightly bent, punch forward like you're knockin' out those bullies who always made mean comments about you, finishing with your left foot and left fist forward.

3. Jump, switch your feet, and punch forward with your right fist, like you're knocking out all those bad food choices you've made in the past. Repeat 10 times. We are well on our way to knocking out that old, unhealthy lifestyle!

X-Hops

To get ready for this activity, either draw or use tape to form an *X* on the ground. This drill is a little more challenging than the first three. When you master it, you should feel a sense of accomplishment and your mood should turn from frustrated to hoppy. (Sorry, I had to!)

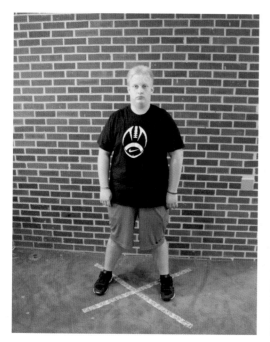 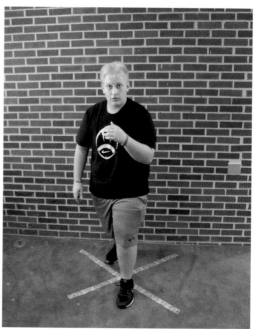

1. Start with your hands by your sides and your feet shoulder-width apart, one on the right side of the *X* and one on the left side.

2. Jump up and swing one foot in front of the other, to the front and back of the *X*.

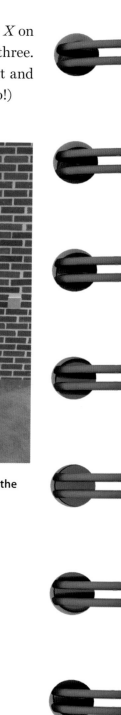

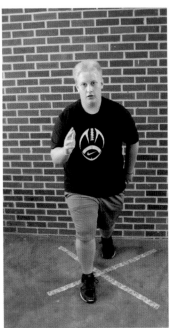
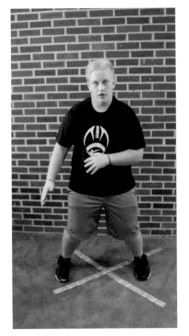
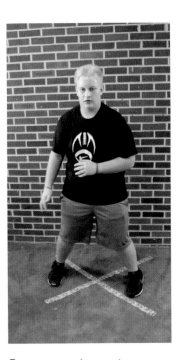

3. Jump again to return your feet to the starting position.

4. Jump again, swinging your feet opposite from last time.

5. Return to the starting position. Keep it up for 30 seconds! Repeat 9 times for a set of 10.

Wall Reaction Drill

You know why we do this drill, right? Two words: Wall Ball!

This drill will improve your reaction time as it gets you moving. You'll need a partner.

1. Stand in a ready position several feet from a wall, facing the wall. Have someone stand behind you with 2 tennis balls.

2. Have your partner throw one ball against the wall to your right. Catch it as it bounces off the wall. Then have your partner throw the second ball against the wall to your left. Since you're pretty close to the wall, if you don't catch the balls, odds are they're going to go past you. That's okay. If you miss one, just keep going with the other ball. (Come on—really run for those balls!)

3. Throw the balls back to your partner to continue the drill. Try to either catch 10 in a row or continue catching until you have dropped both balls and they have bounced by you. Then hustle to pick them up and start over.

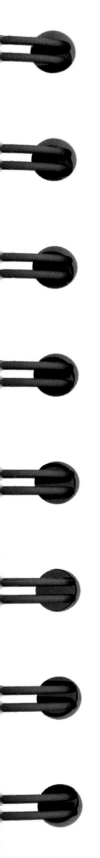
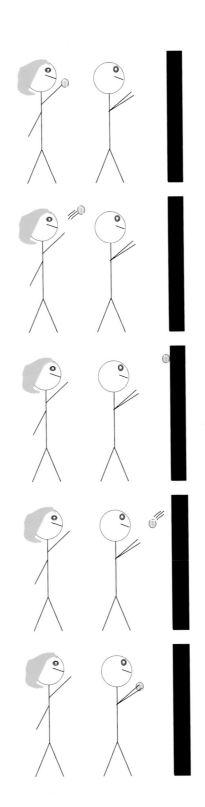

Get into WiiHab!

When I give talks to kids, I always mention that we need to get off the video games. But I don't mean all video games. What I'm saying is, what's the point of sitting on a couch using just your thumbs when you can be up and moving your whole body?

I know a lot of you out there really love your video games and that you have your favorites, whether they're based on your favorite book, movie, or sport. Playing a sitting game is fine every now and then. But do you have any that you have to stand up to play?

I do, and they're my favorites. The great thing about these games is that when I play with my friends, we are all so competitive that we never sit down! We're always bouncing around the room, cheering on our team or whoever is playing at the time.

Below is a list of some of my favorite active video games. All of them are loads of fun and will keep you moving when it's raining out or when you're stuck at home all day.

- *Wii Fit*
- *Dance Central*
- *NFL Training Camp*
- *Motion Sports*
- *Tiger Woods PGA Tour*
- *Wii Sports*
- *Madden NFL & NCAA Football*

If you've never played any of these active games, now's the time to try one! Maybe you can find one that allows you to try an activity you've always wanted to try, like tennis, yoga, dancing, boxing, baseball, or martial arts. If it's active and you're into it, chances are it's been turned into a game!

I hope "WiiHab" turns out to be just as much fun for you as it is for me! It just goes to show you that you can be active every day whether you're in the real world or in the virtual world!

CHAPTER 9

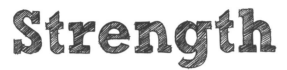

Strong like a Bull

I was maybe a year old, and Mom and Dad put me in one of those saucers on wheels that are supposed to help babies learn to walk. After I cruised a few laps, they took me out and laid me next to it to watch a football game (Florida State University, I hope) and went to get something to drink. When they came back, I was lifting that saucer up and down over my head. Baby bench presses! Dad was so proud—it was time to alert the pro scouts.

Strength is a funny topic for big kids like us. Because we are bigger than most, people sometimes assume we are stronger than most. But I know that when it came to doing push-ups and pull-ups, I felt like the weakest kid in the world. Having to try to pull or push my body when I was at my higher weights was very humbling.

I knew that building up my strength would help me in all aspects of my journey, and it has. And it will help you in yours too, whether you're a girl or a guy. Strong kids don't get bullied, and once

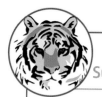

From: Kaila
Subject: Team Tiger Member

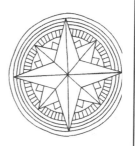

I'm Tiger's favorite sister (okay, I'm his only sister), Kaila, and I'm eleven years old. And I want you to know how many of my friends, girls at school, and girls at the camps and speeches Tiger does, have had their lives changed by Team Tiger—I think we have more girl Team Tiger members than boys.

Now, by the time you're reading this book, you know all about Tiger and my family, but I'm here to tell you a little about me. I'm a cheerleader for Tiger's football teams, and I am the only girl in my family, so you may know how that feels. I have three brothers: Tiger, Zack, and Mike. What I have learned is that you can't be on your own on your journey. You need a team (your family) behind you cheering you on. Sometimes it just needs a sprinkle of girl power and it will blow up!!

Team Tiger is not just for boys. It is totally for girls too. I mean, who says girls can't be involved with football? Whoever said that was cray cray! Don't listen to people who say, "Oh, you can't do it," or "You're not good enough." All you got to do is turn around and say, "Watch me." Just remember, don't ever let anyone bully you or another person! The one thing I know is the bullies are the weak ones. The strong ones are the ones like you who are willing to make a change.

Now, if your brother is practicing for football, how do you keep active? Every single practice, I'm there warming up with them, and when the practice starts, I go walk with other sisters or we practice cheering or even go to the park and walk around. So just remember, you're not alone or left out—you've just got to be creative and find fun ways to keep moving.

Let's try this one more time. My name is Kaila Greene, and my life is about being part of a team. So welcome to Team Tiger, and remember—girls rule!!

you're strong, you can protect other kids from the bullies who used to bother you. Being strong makes working out easier. You take some strain off your back and joints because building up muscle helps support joints and adds stability. I also knew that getting stronger would help me in football. (I know, I know, I mention football a lot. But I really love football!)

When you think of strength training, maybe you picture dumbbells, barbells, or weight-training machines. But did you know that you can use your own body weight to strengthen your muscles? That's what you'll be doing in the exercises below. You don't need to belong to a gym or buy any special equipment to do them. These five exercises work all the big muscles in your body, including your stomach (abdominals, or abs), back, legs, chest, and shoulders, and they will improve your muscle strength and endurance just as well as any exercise you can do in the gym.

A rep is lifting and lowering a weight—in this case, your body—one time. A set is a group of reps. To start, try to do one set of ten reps. If you can't get to ten, do as many as you can with good form. By good form, I mean doing the exercise slowly and with focus, so that you can feel the particular muscle group being used in that activity. Just rushing to get through the repetitions won't achieve the results you want. This is a marathon, not a sprint. If you keep at it, your muscles will get stronger and you'll be able to increase the number of reps and sets you do.

As your strength improves, work up to three to five sets of ten reps. Listen to your body, and pay attention to your form. Doing ten reps right is better than doing twenty reps with sloppy form. Work at your own pace, but do work—you have to start where you are, but you can build from there.

One cool thing about adding strength and muscle is that muscle burns a whole lot more calories than fat does and so helps with weight loss. Remember, though, that muscle weighs more than fat, so the scale isn't always the best guide to your progress. You can track it just by looking in the mirror. The smaller sizes you'll soon be wearing are a pretty good indicator of success too!

Crunches

I've never been good at sit-ups, but crunches are doable, even for big kids. You're not trying to lift your whole body to your knees, and crunches don't hurt your neck. Make sure to keep your ab muscles and stomach tight while you do these. And, just because you can, knock out a few during commercials when you're watching TV.

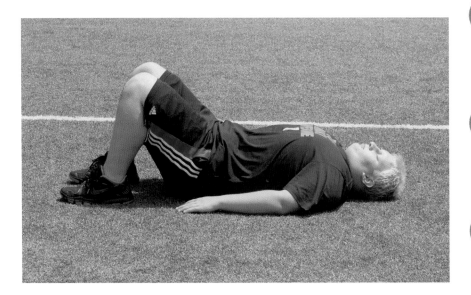

1. Lie on your back on a carpeted floor or a mat. Bend your knees, place your feet a little less than shoulder-width apart, put your arms by your sides, and tighten your abdominal muscles.

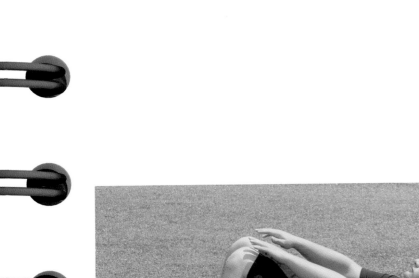

2. Using your abs, slowly raise your upper body as far as you can, reaching toward your knees with your hands. Then lower yourself back to the mat. Do 9 more repetitions to complete a set of 10.

Planks

In the beginning I found these tough—my stomach was in the way! But I kept doing the best I could, and soon enough, planks were a walk in the park—not a bad idea for after your workout. (If you're doing these on concrete or turf in the summer heat, use a towel or a mat. Once I actually burned my forearms doing this!)

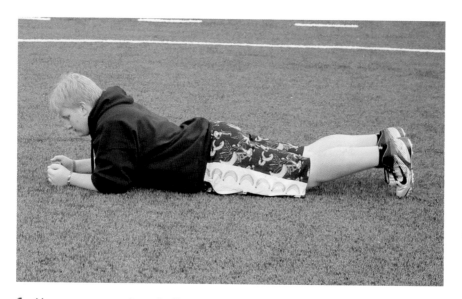

1. Lie on your stomach on the floor or ground with your elbows bent, your forearms straight out in front of you, and your knees slightly bent. Keep your toes on the ground so your calves are slightly elevated.

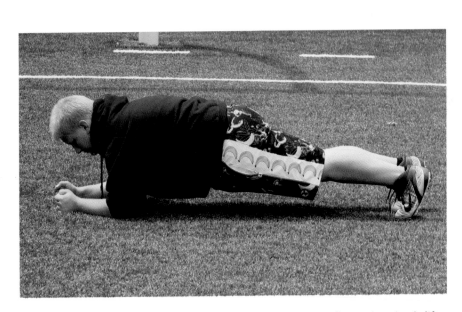

2. Pushing up on your forearms while tightening your stomach muscles, slowly lift your body so that only your forearms and toes are touching the ground. Keep your back as straight as possible. Hold for 30 seconds. Then slowly lower your body back to the starting position. Repeat 9 more times for a set of 10.

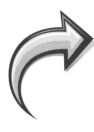

Squats

Big kids like us can usually do squats really well. Because our legs are used to carrying our body weight, they are usually the strongest part of our bodies. (Finally, some good news.)

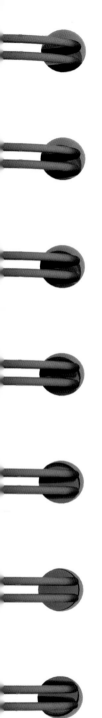

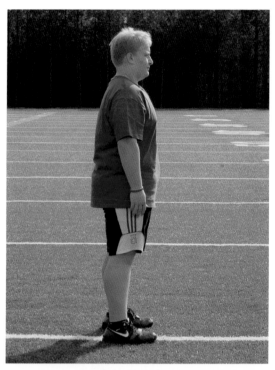

1. Stand with your feet shoulder-width apart, knees slightly bent, back straight, and your arms by your side.

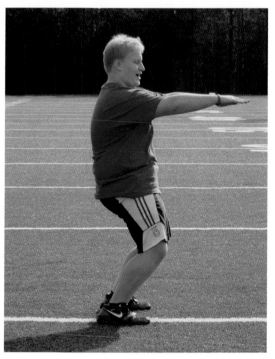

2. Extend your arms straight out in front of you and slowly bend your knees more, as if you were about to sit down in a chair, until you feel a slight burn in your legs. Keep your back as straight as you can and make sure that your knees do not move past your toes. Hold this position for 30 seconds and then return to a standing position. Repeat 9 more times for a set of 10.

David's Story

Weighing over five hundred pounds, David was the largest kid at our camp, and his mom was even bigger. They arrived late, and it took them a while to get down the dome's seventy-two steps. But the fact that he made it to the camp at all from his home in southern Georgia proved that David was determined to change.

When I met him, the look in his eyes and his slumped shoulders told me that he wasn't real sure about what he'd gotten himself into. So while Dad gave him one of those pep talks I knew so well from our football games, I went to find Marcus and Mike Peterson—a linebacker and, like Marcus, an outgoing, positive guy. I figured meeting those guys could definitely offer David a little extra inspiration!

David's face lit up as he saw these two very big dudes, all suited up, approaching. "Every dream—whether it's to play in the NFL or just to get healthier—has a starting point," I remember Mike saying to David. "This is yours."

While Mike and I walked David to Dr. Craighead's group, Dad headed in the opposite direction—toward David's mother, who had gone to watch the camp from the seats. Okay, that wasn't gonna happen. No one sits and watches at a Team Tiger camp! It's all about getting involved, seizing the moment, and making it your own. Although we big kids have to take responsibility for ourselves, we need our team—our friends and family—to support us on our journeys.

Fortunately, David's mother rose to the challenge. She spent the rest of the camp by David's side, going through the stations with him. He did awesome and took part in everything we did. At one of the first stations, he kept letting kids get in front of him. I suspected he was nervous about doing the drill, which required him to lift his knees high.

"We'll do this one side by side," I told him, and we did, with Mike cheering him on. He completed the whole drill—sweaty, winded, but with an ear-to-ear grin. I knew what he was feeling: pride.

I kind of trailed him all over the camp, but by the last station, he waved me off. "I got this," he said, and he did.

As the camp ended, my mom noticed a young man sitting near where Shane had set up his station in the end zone. (I didn't see this—I was somewhere else, saying my good-byes.) It took a minute for her to realize it was David eating from a giant pan of ribs and fries. Hungry after an activity-fueled day, he had ripped into one of the "what not to order" displays Shane had set up. "I didn't know whether to laugh or cry," she said later.

Thankfully, that's not the end of the story. Dad and I had connected David and his mom with every expert in this book, and we followed up with phone calls for months. Eating right and exercising daily—either walking or following the work-outs we'd given him—he ended up losing sixty pounds, and his mother lost fifty.

Yes, they worked out and ate right together—a little team of two, connected to a larger team they'd met at our camp. It just goes to show that when you don't give up, good things can happen.

David has promised me he'll be at the next camp at the dome so he can help lead one of the groups. I can't wait to see him.

Triceps Dips

I'm not gonna lie—while big kids' legs are strong, our upper bodies usually aren't. So triceps dips aren't easy at first. But keep doing them, because sooner than you think, you'll be ready to tackle that rock-climbing wall at the theme park or gym!

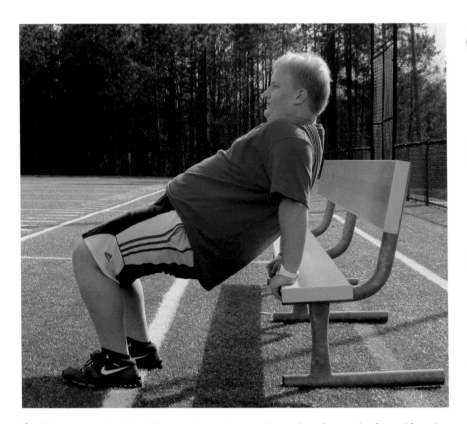

1. Sit on a sturdy chair with your knees bent and your feet flat on the floor. (If you're doing this exercise outside, you can use a park bench or a curb.) Place your hands next to your hips and grasp the edge of the chair. Lift up onto your hands and bring your hips forward.

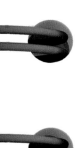

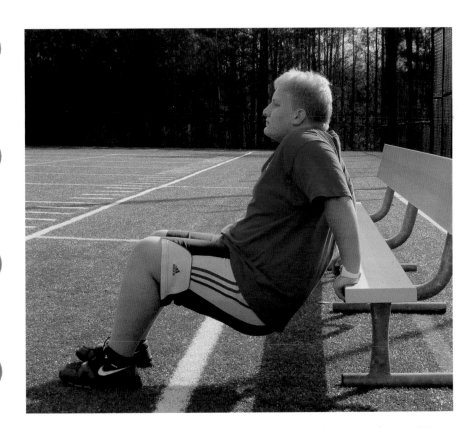

2. Lower your hips toward the floor until your elbows are bent to 90 degrees. Keep your hips close to the chair and your shoulders down. Without locking your elbows, push back up through your palms until your arms are straight. Return to the starting position and do 9 more repetitions to complete the set of 10.

Push-Ups

If you're anything like I was (heavy and weak in the upper body), you'll want to start with a modified push-up, which you do on your knees—and that's okay. Just keep adding one or two reps to your sets every week. Once your upper body gets stronger, you'll be able to do full-on push-ups, like I do now.

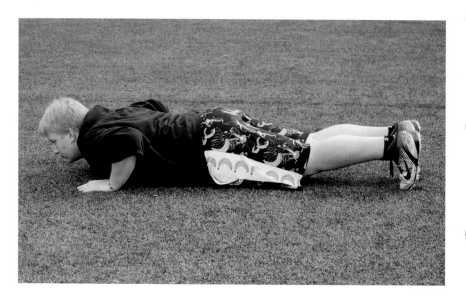

1. Lie facedown on the ground or mat with your hands positioned directly under your shoulders and dig your toes into the ground or mat. Your whole body should touch the surface except for your shins.

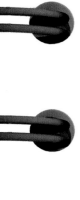

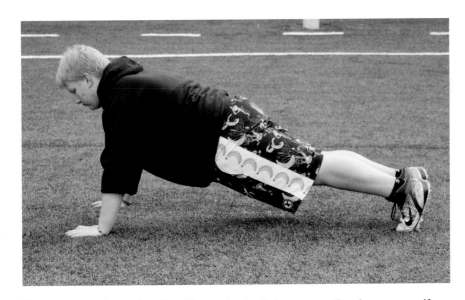

2. Push through your hands to lift your body all the way up. Then lower yourself until your arms are bent at a 90-degree angle. Repeat 9 more times and try to add one more each day! Try to go a little lower each week until eventually you can touch the ground with your chest. (My brother Zack does, like, 50 of these, and I just want to go and sit on him!)

Kickin' It—Cardio That's Cool

My favorite video dance game is *Dance Central*. Zack, Kaila, and I love to play it with our favorite babysitter, Sarah, for hours. Kaila actually sets up date nights for Mom and Dad just so we can have Sarah over and get our dance contest going. I may not have rhythm, but I do have fun.

Between dance offs, you can keep moving by loading your iPod with upbeat tunes. Even if you're riding in the car, walking to school, or just kickin' it with friends, you'll keep some bounce in your step. Here are twelve of my favorite "kickin' it" tunes:

1. "Evacuate the Dance Floor" (Cascada)
2. "Cupid Shuffle" (Cupid)
3. "Poker Face" (Lady Gaga)
4. "Dynamite" (Taio Cruz)
5. "I Gotta Feeling" (Black-Eyed Peas)
6. "Whip My Hair" (Willow Smith)
7. "U Can't Touch This" (MC Hammer)
8. "Cha Cha Slide" (Mr. C the Slide Man)
9. "Cheeseburger in Paradise" (Jimmy Buffett)
10. "Live Those Songs" (Kenny Chesney)
11. "The Boys of Fall" (Kenny Chesney)

And last, but not least. . .

12. "Eye of the Tiger" (Survivor)

Add your own, and let's see you bust a move!

If you really like to dance, ask your mom or dad to see about signing you up for some type of dance class. Since all these dancing shows hit TV, classes are everywhere, including at your local gym, YMCA, or YWCA.

CHAPTER 10

Flexibility

Loosen Up!

When I was heavier, my joints and muscles ached all the time. Carrying a lot of extra weight is tough on the back, knees, and ankles— maybe you can relate. No wonder I never wanted to work out! Doing the simplest things seemed impossible, and I'm not even talking about exercise. I'd drop a pencil on the floor, and instead of bending over to pick it up, I would think up an excuse as to why I didn't need it. (On second thought, since I got a C on my algebra test with that pencil, I'm just gonna leave it on the floor.)

There are no excuses for not being flexible—kids are supposed to be limber! While you may not have given any thought to flexibility, it's an important part of being fit and healthy. Loose, flexible muscles and joints make it easier to move— you won't hurt anymore, and you'll be more and more able to do the fun stuff you want to do. Or even just the basic stuff. As silly as this sounds, as I lost weight and my flexibility improved, bending over to tie my shoes became a pretty big accomplishment in my mind. No one but you needs to know that—but come on, it would be cool to be able to scratch an itch on your back. Am I right? And soon enough I went from sitting cross-legged—a feat in itself—to running in my second 10K Peachtree Road Race and swimming and working out later the same day.

The flexibility exercises below will take less than five minutes of each of your workouts, but they're important minutes, so don't blow them off! If you're gonna do something, do it with heart! So as you go through the exercises in this station, keep these points in mind.

Start each stretch slowly, exhaling as you gently stretch the muscle. Seriously, be gentle. And don't bounce when you stretch because that can injure your muscles. Stretching shouldn't hurt either. If you feel pain, you've stretched too far.

Try to hold each stretch for thirty seconds, and breathe deeply and evenly as you stretch. Use your stretching time to chill out and listen to your body. Although your main goal here is to increase the flexibility of your muscles, you just may find that doing these exercises relaxes your mind and reduces your stress too!

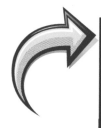

Coach Z's Top Tips

- If you start to cramp during any stretch or exercise, slowly stretch the cramp, but do not stretch it aggressively. If it persists, use ice to massage it, rubbing slowly on the cramped muscle to help it relax. (Never ice any muscle longer than twenty minutes.)

- Do these flexibility exercises any time you're just hanging out—sitting at your computer, playing video games, watching TV, or texting your friends. They're great to do as a break from homework too! Make it a habit to get up and move every half hour or so. As you get into your new routine, get moving during commercials and enjoy some WiiHab!

A Tiger Tale

When I think of my newfound fitness, a football story comes to mind (of course). Remember my dog Scout? Well, one of his many nicknames is Bulldozer. He is very jealous and can't stand it when we pay attention to one of our other pets, so he bulldozes in between us and the cat or our other dog, Sakki, and you can't get around him.

When Dad realized how much strength and quickness I had gained, he was inspired to create a new play for our team called the Bulldozer Wedge. For you football folks, it's a glorified QB sneak behind me as center. For those of you who don't speak football, it's a play where basically our quarterback gets the ball from me and then grabs my jersey, tucks himself behind me, and follows me as far as he can. (You guessed it—I am the bulldozer.)

We once ran the Bulldozer Wedge eight plays in a row—ninety yards for a touchdown. The other coach was so frustrated that he had four guys try to stop me on every play after that. But there is no stopping the bulldozer, and we ran it successfully the rest of the game. I don't like the thought of you "bulldozing" in front of people in public and being rude, but you may be able to get past your brother or sister to have first dibs at the fruit salad!

Chest/Shoulder Stretch

This stretch feels awesome—I just did it, as I was writing this, to take a break. It's amazing how stretching can loosen you up both physically and mentally.

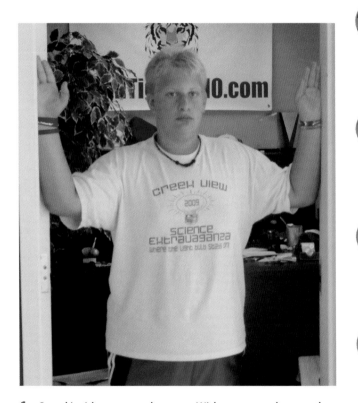

1. Stand inside an open doorway. With your arms bent at the elbows, place your forearms on both sides of the doorway. (If you're outdoors, place one arm on the side of a pole or tree.)

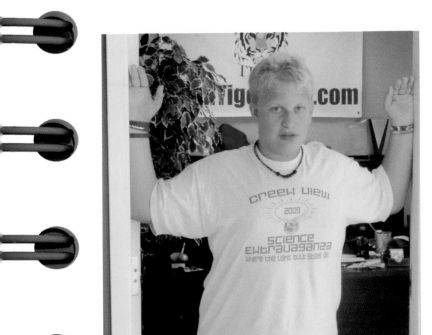

2. Gently lean forward, letting your body weight come forward. You will feel a slight stretch across your chest and shoulder area, and your shoulders will kind of pinch together behind you. Hold the stretch for 30 seconds and then slowly return to the starting position. Repeat 3 to 5 times.

Calf Stretch

After doing this stretch for a few days, start to take small steps away from the wall to increase the stretch a little. Remember to keep your feet flat and to slowly walk toward the wall to end the stretch.

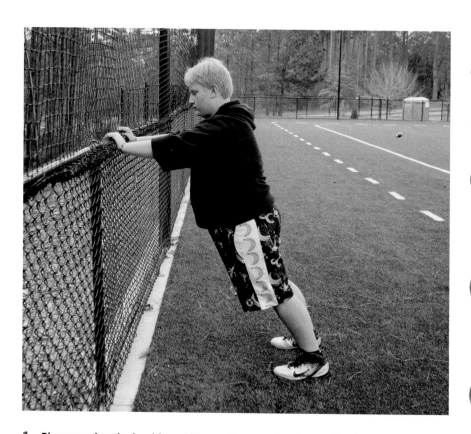

1. Place your hands shoulder-width apart on a wall or fence. Slowly walk backward until your feet are about 2 feet from the wall or fence, and place them shoulder-width apart.

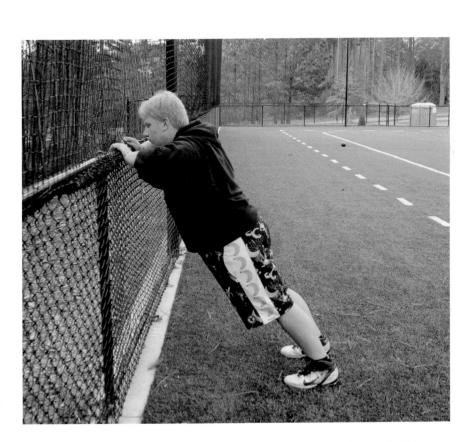

2. Bend your arms slowly, keeping your heels flat on the ground so you feel the stretch. Slowly return to the starting position. Repeat 3 to 5 times.

Hip Flexor Stretch

The hip flexors are a group of muscles that lift the knee upward when you walk and run. It is very important for me to get this part of my body loose, or else I'll be as slow as the old Tiger felt waiting on his cheesesteak.

This stretch may seem a little boring, but—like homework and broccoli—sometimes boring stuff brings good results.

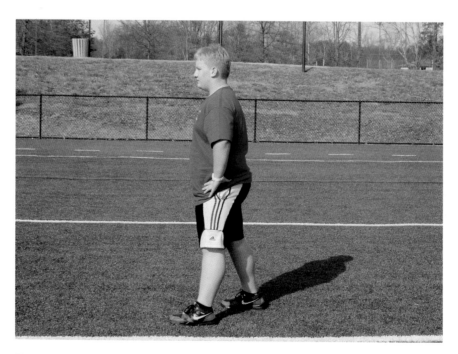

1. Stand tall with your hands on your hips, like your mom does when she's mad at you. This gives you good balance. Place one foot in front of the other with your toes pointed forward.

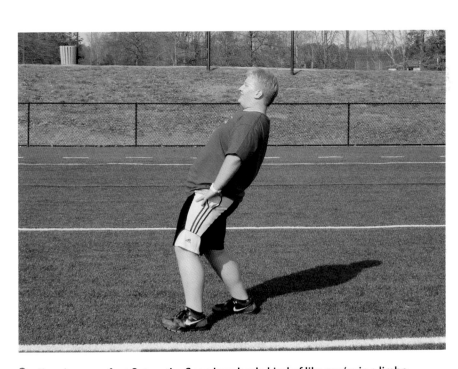

2. Keeping your feet flat on the floor, lean back, kind of like you're in a limbo contest, until you feel a mild stretch in your back leg on the front of your thigh. Keep your balance, and don't lean back so much that your back hurts or twinges. Hold the stretch for 30 seconds, and then repeat on your other leg. Repeat 3 to 5 times with each leg.

Quad Stretch

The muscles on the front of your thighs, the quadriceps (quads for short), are some of the largest muscles in your body. So strengthening them and improving their flexibility adds a lot to your core strength and base (a term for some of the body's largest muscle groups, particularly your legs and abdomen). Your base is like the foundation of a building. Having a strong base supports everything else and gives you something to build on.

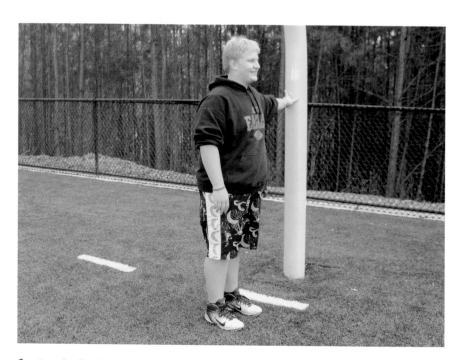

1. Stand tall with your feet slightly apart, your right hand down by your side, and your left stretched out to your support (like a goalpost, wall, or fence) or just in the air to help you balance.

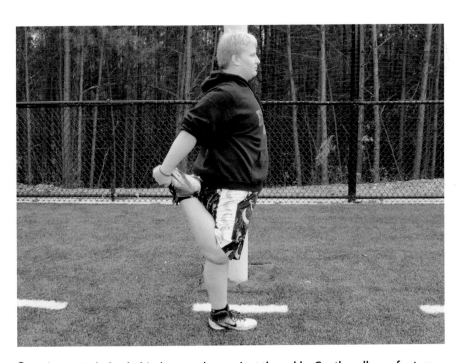

2. Lift your right leg behind you and grasp it at the ankle. Gently pull your foot up toward your butt until you feel a mild stretch in your thigh. Your thigh should be pulled straight back; don't let it wander to the side! Hold this position for 30 seconds and then repeat with your left leg. Repeat 3 to 5 times with each leg. Again, do not be overly aggressive at first—stretch only as far as you feel comfortable. Then, try to increase that range a little more each day. Remember that do-a-little-better-each-day thing I told you about a few pages back?

Hamstring Stretch

Now you'll stretch the muscles on the back of your thighs, called the hamstrings. It's really important to stretch your hammies, and it also feels really good when you're done. The nice thing about your hammies is that they'll definitely let you know if you're stretching them too far. (Mine hurt a little bit today after conditioning yesterday—but in a good way!)

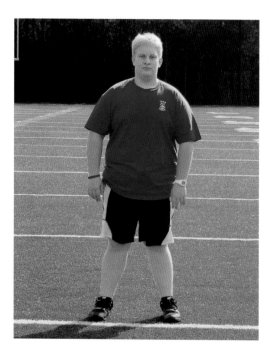

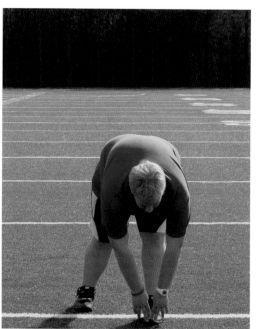

1. Stand tall with your hands at your sides and your feet shoulder-width apart.

2. Place one foot in front of the other and then slowly bend forward from your hips to reach as far down toward your front foot as you can. Keep your balance and go at your own pace. Don't overextend; always go slow and easy and let your body guide you.

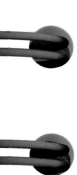

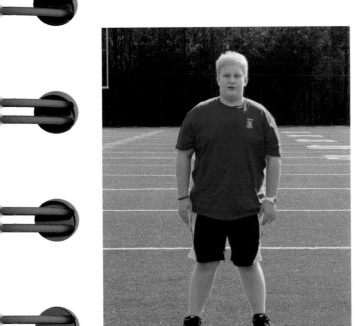
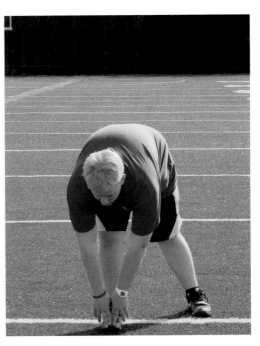

3. Hold the stretch for 30 seconds and then return to the starting position.

4. Repeat with your other leg in front. Do this 3 to 5 times for each leg.

Championship Golf:
From (Tiger) Greene to the Green

I used to think that cardio was supposed to be me dragging my big behind on a treadmill till I was so exhausted I couldn't keep up and went flying off the back into a wall. But I couldn't write a whole book without mentioning cardio, Tiger-style. It's called golf.

According to Coach Z, I'm supposed to keep my heart rate up for a certain period of time. I try to do it every day. And the way I figure it, any cardio is better than none, so when I started my journey, I decided to take advantage of the spring weather and find an outdoor activity that I enjoyed: I tried golf to get the ball rolling (kind of a golf joke). Today, I love golf almost as much as I love football.

Golf got me to start taking pride in my appearance—off came the big, baggy, hide-my-tummy clothes. One of the reasons I stopped playing baseball (besides not being very good at it) was that I hated the tight uniforms—they never had my size. I always felt like baseball was not meant for big kids—or, at least, not me.

These days, my golf outfit usually involves looking like a human flag, complete with star-studded USA flag belt buckle. Or I mix and match bright colors and wild patterns to produce an outfit that only I and Stevie Wonder could love (who gave one of the best concerts I've ever been to, by the way). Then I surprised my parents and golf pros and told them I didn't need a cart; I was gonna walk (Dad was smiling but starting to sweat already). It really wasn't as big of a change as Dad thought it would be because when you factor in all of the walking he does, looking in the woods and sand traps and creeks for his ball, he's usually worn out by the time he gets back to the cart anyway.

Golf can be a good workout if you walk the course, which I do whenever they allow it (although sometimes it's too busy). Even though we stop to hit shots, we're still walking distances while we enjoy our family and friends and the fresh air. We have a blast! As we finish the eighteenth hole, we make sure to let everyone know that we just walked almost five miles. (Boy, you would think golfers would be too tired to go out and get into trouble after that workout. That must be why they drive their SUVs into trees.)

So, if you're able, you might want to give golf a shot. Even if you have to take a cart, you can still walk every hole after your tee shot and get almost the same distance out of your day. I remember the first time I walked the course with a friend. He was huffing and puffing after a few holes, so we only played a few. The next time we played, it became a few more than nine. After a few weeks of joining me in my other activities, he was better conditioned. Then each time we got together, he could do a little more cardio, even if it was just a few more holes.

Like all other exercise, you can golf at your own pace, build up as slowly as you wish, and enjoy the game and your progress. While you may never have played golf, it's fun to try to use your cardio, flexibility, and strength. (And if you're playing with my Uncle Larry, you'll also use your agility and quickness to get out of the way of his sideways shots!) If you check at your local public courses, they have kids' rates and clubs—you might be able to play after school for as little as ten dollars, and it might even be free with some other programs that the PGA sponsors.

It's time to grip it and rip it!

A Tiger Tale

I know we bring some things upon ourselves, and part of empowering ourselves on this journey is realizing where we've gone wrong in the past. So when I started thinking about how important flexibility is, I immediately had a flashback to the first time Coach Z and Mom made me take a yoga class at the beginning of my journey.

Rule numero uno: never eat Mexican food before your first yoga class. It's a really bad idea—mostly for those around you. My Barking Dog pose—that's what I call it—brought tears to everyone's eyes, and I don't think they were tears of pride or joy. I know that a lot of athletes and people in general have turned to yoga to improve their flexibility, but I prefer standard flexibility exercises not named after animals. Also—and this is a personal thing—I like to keep my face out of the general direction of people's lower bodies while they're wearing tight pants.

The End (of This Book, Not Your Journey)

This last chapter marks the official beginning of your journey, which is a big deal. Every journey should have a huge send-off. I wish I could end this book like I end our Team Tiger camps.

If it was up to me, you and your parents, and hundreds of other kids and their parents, would be gathering around the stage in the middle of the field. The speakers would erupt with the Black Eyed Peas' "I Gotta Feeling." Marcus, some of our cheerleaders, Zack, Kaila, and I would be on the stage leading a giant flash mob dance, and you'd be dancing along with us. The lyrics of that song say it all: "Tonight's gonna be a good, good night." But forget *good* and forget *night*—we're sending you off with the knowledge that it's gonna be a great, great life!

Having read this book, you're ready to go. Hopefully, the resources I've shared with you have started you toward a healthier and more active lifestyle that has no ends or limits. The most important thing I want you to take away from my story is that life isn't about being perfect. It's about getting up each day and doing just a little bit better than the day before. It's about knowing that you're not alone—you're part of my team. And if you play every play and play with heart, you will be a champion in every aspect of your life.

This book is just the beginning of so much more than losing weight. On your journey, you'll also find health, happiness, and inspiration. But most of all, as you start to believe more in yourself, you'll be amazed at the team that starts to build around you and the changes you can make in others. Keep Team Tiger in your heart and in your mind whenever times get tough, because you're not alone. And always remember to look at life and its opportunities through the eyes of a Tiger.

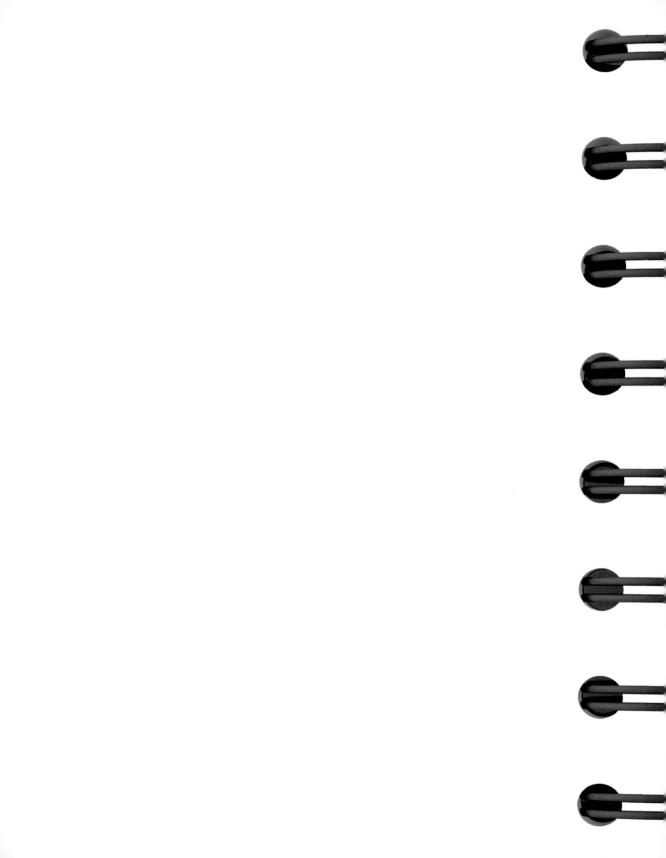

Epilogue

So here we are at the end of this book and, for me, the end of an era. On December 3, 2011, two years after I began my journey, I played my last game with Alpharetta Youth Football—the All-Star game, always the last of the season.

You might remember another All-Star game I mentioned, back in Chapter 2. At that 2009 game, I weighed in at two hundred fifty pounds, my top weight ever. Two weeks after that game, I had my aha moment, formed Team Tiger, and began thinking about writing this book.

What a difference two years makes. At this season's All-Star game, I am in the best shape of my life. I'm fit and completely healthy (no more diabetes or thyroid pills!), and I ran for five touchdowns this season, passed for two, kicked an extra point, caught a couple of passes, and had the season of a lifetime.

I'm sad to see the season go, as this is the last year that my dad will coach me because I move on to high school next year. Even though it's kind of sad, I look forward to the new tasks ahead and the obstacles I am ready to overcome. I want to thank my family, team, and coaches for all the great memories that we made; I appreciate every single moment of our time together. Next year, I get to help Dad coach Zack's team. So get ready, Zack—here I come!

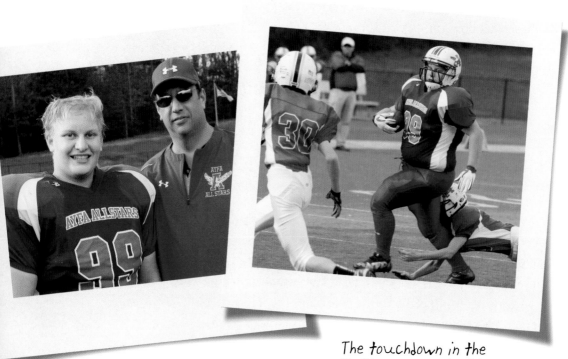

Dad and me after our last game together, the 2011 AYFA All-Star game.

The touchdown in the All-Star game! Nothin' was gonna stop me!

But back to the All-Star game. It got me thinking about how I wanted to end this book. Which means, of course, that I gotta talk football.

But bear with me. This epilogue is about more than a football game. It's about life—and about family. So as Dad might say, take a knee.

The first thing you need to know about this game: Remember that coach who called me a glob? This year, the Greene Machine played against that same coach and his son. Crazy, right? Nope—it was awesome. Because shortly after he called me a glob, those guys became our good friends and huge Team Tiger supporters. When you play with heart, good things happen.

The second thing you need to know: we lost. By halftime, the Greene Machine was down, 19–0. Dad brought us into a huddle for our half-time talk. Before he began, he found me in the huddle and caught my eye, as he always does. I nodded, as I always do. He began to speak. I was pretty sure of what he'd say, and he said it.

"I'm proud of you for making it to the All-Stars after such a great season," he said. "The difference on the scoreboard is just a few plays. Don't look back. As long as we learned from the first half and make the changes we need to make, all that matters is that we go forward. Now go out there and win that second half!"

Now, when Dad says "win," he means, "Give it everything you have, play every play, play four quarters, play as a team, and most of all play with heart." (Now, where have you heard that before?)

Pumped after Dad's halftime talk, we took it to the Red All-Stars (we were the Blue All-Stars—pretty creative, huh?) in the second half. Early on, the ref threw out one of their players for repeated personal

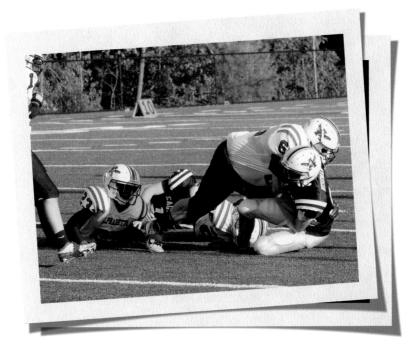

Tackle in the backfield!

fouls. (Funny how bullies usually end up watching the game from the sidelines.)

When we got the ball and were driving for our first touchdown, my teammate told my dad, "Coach, put Tiger and me in the backfield. We will get it to the end zone!" Smiling, Dad nodded and sent us onto the field.

Our center snapped the ball. Just as I got the handoff, someone grabbed my arm, and I fumbled. There was a huge pile on the field. Forget the extra fifty or sixty pounds I used to carry. I now had about eight hundred pounds of kids on me!

After a mad scramble for the ball, the referee pulled us apart. "Red ball!" he shouted.

If that had happened two years ago, I probably would have mentally checked out. But that was then. My teammates helped me up from the pile, and the defense came out to join me. We were gonna get that ball back. In four plays, we did.

"Do you want to swap back to the line?" Dad asked me. Basically, he was asking me if I wanted a safer, out-of-the-spotlight position where I wouldn't have to carry the ball.

I shook my head. "I want the ball," I said. "I'll get us to the end zone."

He nodded. I went to the huddle and called the play.

I think every player, coach, and fan knew I was getting the ball—when I'm in the backfield, I'm gonna run the ball. But it didn't matter. This time I got the handoff, my lead blocker blasted a hole, and I broke one tackle and drove through the rest of the tacklers into the end zone for a touchdown.

I was about to do my touchdown dance when out of nowhere, I was flat on my back. A kid from the other team had hit me with a cheap shot, but then all I saw for those few seconds was the penalty flag waving. My teammates helped me up, and we went on to score again.

We lost the game, 25–12, but we won the second half, just as Dad had told us to do.

Now that I think about it, that last game ties in with the way I think about life—and the way you might think about yours. It doesn't mat-

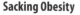

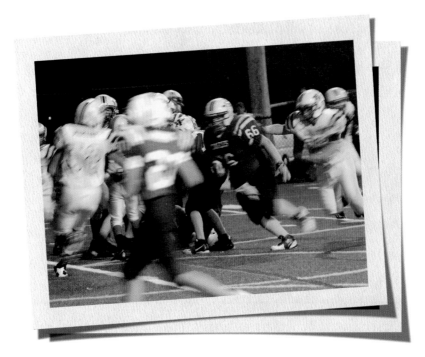

My first touchdown ever on September 24, 2011. My fourteenth birthday!

ter what has happened in your life up until now. That's your first half. You can learn from it. Now, with the right plays and adjustments—the ones you have in this book—you can win your second half. You can change your life from this point forward. You may still have to deal with cheap shots—nasty comments, whispers, stuff like that—like I did in the game (and for most of my life). But as long as you know you are on the right path and doing the right things, you'll win that second half. I've learned that life has a way of taking care of bullies and rewarding those with heart.

I'm lucky to be surrounded with a lot of heart. A lot of my teammates this year made the All-Star team because of it! Emmett, who was our running back this year, had never played in the backfield before, but through determination and dedication, he wound up getting four interceptions and three touchdowns against the number-one team in the play-offs! Another example of heart was our quarterback/kicker

Danny, who on and off the field shows what true heart and friendship is about. He even wrote a school paper about how everything we learn as a team applies to life. And my friend Matt always had my back on the field.

And then there's Mikey—he's #25 in the picture below. His nickname is Small But Mighty, and boy, is he ever. He made the All-Star team because he played every play, every quarter. Giving up never even enters his mind. On or off the field, he's got your back. Mikey and I had different challenges, but both of us learned, early on, to turn obstacles into opportunities. You can too.

When my dad first signed me up for football in first grade, I had no idea what I was supposed to be doing. After that first year, he decided I should skip the next year of football and play fall baseball instead. But in third grade, I started to learn the basic rules and what I was

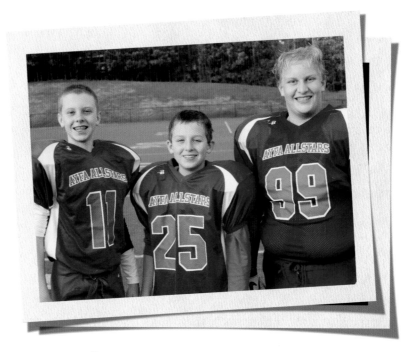

Danny (11), Mikey (25), and me (99)
after the All-Star game.

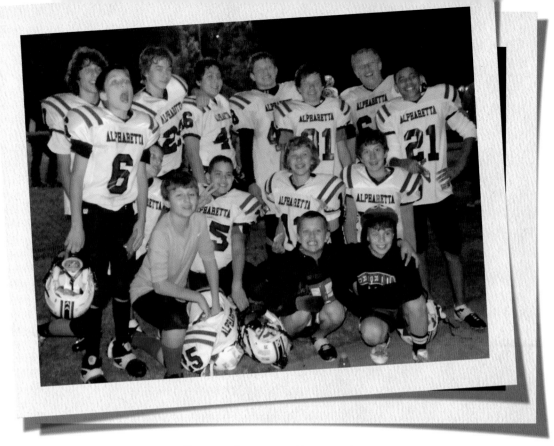

Some of my brothers and me.

out there to do, and I started to enjoy it. I also found out that football is more than what it looks like to the naked eye.

If you haven't played the game, or been around the players on the field, you might watch a game on TV or from the stadium and simply see a bunch of big guys who trash-talk each other and hit people all day long. I'm not saying that stuff doesn't happen because, trust me, it does! But when you play football, you have to depend on your teammates to do their duties and to protect you. In return, you protect them.

Nowhere else in my life had people depended on me like that before. This is why the memories and stories I am most proud of would have to be the ones about my football team/life. Now instead of having two brothers with whom I have a direct family relationship, I have hundreds of brothers that have shed blood with me on the field.

That is why football plays such a big role in my life. It's because football is not just a team, it's not just a season, and it's not just a game. It's a family that stays by your side no matter what and that you depend on to be there with you through thick and thin.

Any members of a sports team can get close to each other. But when it comes to such a rough and physical sport like football, you've got to rely on your brothers. A football team is a family. They might not live with you, and you probably don't look anything like them, but that's what makes it unique. A football team can bring together so many different kinds of people, cultures, and personalities. We may not all look the same—some may be faster than others, some heavier than others—but we are all special in our own way.

I've already hung my last helmet and jersey from the Alpharetta Green Eagles in my basement, with all my others from years past. I have never been more proud. Each piece of equipment holds a special story that helps me reflect on the incredible time my dad and I have had together during my not-so-peewee football years and all that I have overcome and accomplished since then.

I am so blessed that my journey has brought you and me together. Please let me know your successes and let me help with your challenges. Keep in touch at TeamTiger.org.

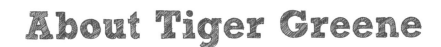

About Tiger Greene

When only 12 years old, Tiger Greene founded a non-profit organization called Team Tiger to help other "big kids" get healthy. Tiger's passion for football drove him to create a relationship with the NFL, who took up the call to help fight against childhood obesity, and Team Tiger soon became a national phenomenon. A media favorite, Tiger has been featured on "The Dr. Oz Show," CNN's "Anderson Cooper 360," and others. As National Ambassador for the NFL Fuel Up to Play 60 program, which represents over 36 million kids and 70,000 schools, Tiger is proud to be able to help kids—and their families—continue on the journey to good health.

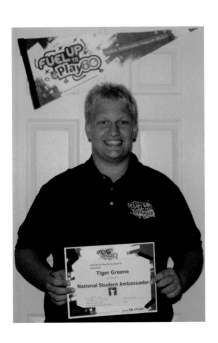

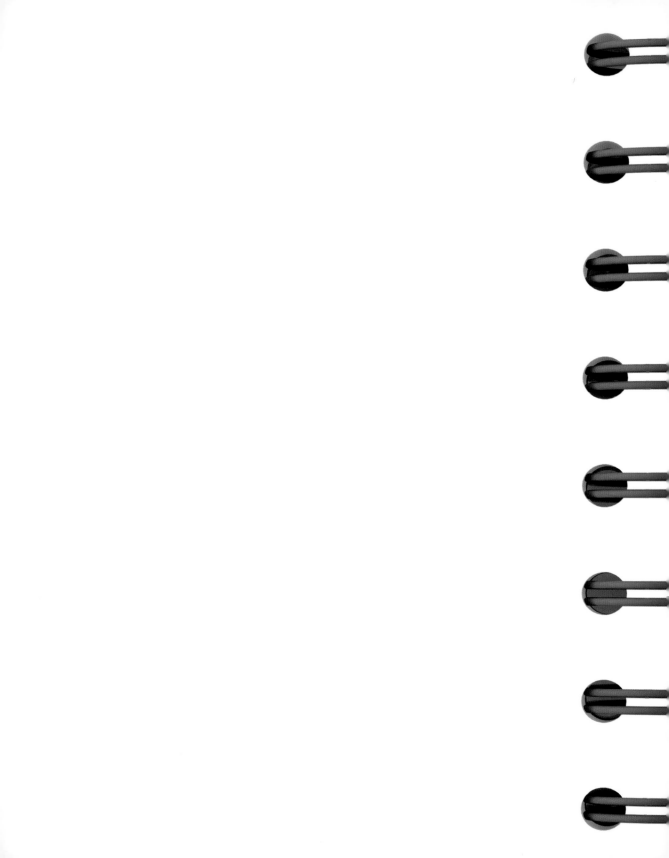

Acknowledgments

There is truly a reason for Team Tiger. The fact is that my journey, transformation, and ability to reach and help kids all over the world is because of the help, support, and love of so many people.

My journey began and will always continue with Coach Z. Ohana Forever, Brah! Then we go on to a few doctors: Dr. Bill Knopf, who saved my dad's life and kick-started my journey; to Dr. Mehmet Oz, who gave us the harsh reality of the path we were on and introduced us to Dr. Linda Craighead, who is Team Tiger's rock; and on to Dr. Gupta, for helping me show kids there is hope. And Dr. Crabtree, Dr. Collier, and Dr. Nick Sudano for all your care, concern, time, and support. To Jeffrey Smith, who believed in my book and got it into the hands of Amy Rennert, who didn't care that I was just twelve years old but was willing to help me tell my story. Then the folks at HarperOne, who were so patient with a kid, but impassioned enough to help me get these resources to you so together we can change the world. Our dear friend Charlie Feehan and his whole family, who, no matter the craziness of their own lives, always made time to support me and our cause, and for getting Shane involved with our camps and foundation. All of Coach Z's folks who ran stations at our camps, including Rob, Timmy, Matt, and all their volunteers—thanks for being ohana. The amazing folks for two years at The Georgia Dome, Levy Food services, and Georgia State University football program, who went way beyond any expectation I could have had to support our Sacking Obesity camps.

Mike, Jeremy, Mark and Scott, Sarah and Jay—you rock!! And most of all, thanks to my partner in Sacking Obesity, Marcus Stroud—you're the real deal, Big Man. To Chuck Smith—thank you for supporting me and pushing me to be the best I can be. Also to Brian Kozlowski and his wife, Ellen; Brian and Erin Finneran; Matt and Sarah Ryan; and Brian Jordan for believing in me and making me feel special way before there was ever Team Tiger. You gave me the courage to believe in myself no matter what I weighed or looked like—you will never know how much that friendship changed my life. Tyler, thank you for stepping into Team Tiger and for all your support. To Matt, Laura, and Kathy at Powerade Zero, your partnership means a lot. To Harry's Farmers Market/Whole Foods for all your support—you're awesome, Jennifer. I can't forget Eileen—a big thx. I want to thank my friend Julia Vantine for helping me get this book done. To Trequita and the whole National Dairy Counsel and the NFL Fuel Up to Play 60 program—thank you for believing me and supporting me and making me National Ambassador. I will work my hardest to make you proud!

By this point I'm sure it's no secret how important my friends and family are to me. To my friend Danny and the entire Cooney clan, I can't ever imagine having a bigger (or louder!) support group. I love you guys but I gotta say it, Go Noles! To Mikey and all the Molinaris, thank you not only for all your support but for your inspiration. You truly are small but mighty! For those times when I feel like just absolutely being a goofball, I know Emmett is always there for me. Thank you and your family for always letting me be myself. To Matt, thanks for always having my back, Brochacho, and I've always got yours! And to Madi, thanks for all the long hours helping out at Team Tiger and, most of all, just for being a great friend. And I know I mentioned the Feehans earlier. But I gotta single out Mark, cause he was always there for me long before my journey started and it's friends like that that make dreams like this possible. IDC, IDK. :)

And again to all those I haven't named but have shown your love and support: I am and always will be forever grateful. I have left so many unnamed—but, I promise, none unappreciated.

Index

Page references followed by *p* indicate a photograph.

ABCs of being a big kid, 65
active video games, 174
activity stations: for agility activities and drills, 137–58; for flexibility activities and drills, 136, 191–206; for quickness activities and drills, 136, 159–74; for strength activities and drills, 136, 175–90; Team Tiger Camp use of, 136
agility activities: Clockwork Drill, 152–53; Cuts Drill, 146–49*p*; importance of developing agility through, 136, 137–38; In-Out Ladder Drill, 154*p*–56*p*; T-Drill, 142–45*p*; Tiger Tail Drill, 140–41
aha moment, 31, 32, 38, 64
Alpharetta Youth Football All-Star game (2009): as closing chapter of my journey, 209–16; Dad and Tiger during the, 210*p*; photographs of the, 210*p*, 211*p*; team members, 214*p*, 215*p*. See

also Green Eagles [Green(e) Machine] football team
arthritis, 65
asthma, 66
Atlanta Falcons, 43–44
Atlanta Little League concession stands, 129–31

barbecue joints, 127
Barking Dog (yoga pose), 206
"Be the tree": as the goal, 16–17; how your family can help you, 19
The Biggest Loser (TV show): lack of inspiration to Tiger, 13, 38–39; resources for contestants, 43; watching the contestants on, 28–29
blaming, 15
bread baskets, 122
breakfast: importance of eating, 59, 77, 92; suggestions for healthy, 93*p*–94*p*
Breast Friends Golf Tournament (2009), 9*p*
Bulldozer Wedge (football play), 35–36*p*, 193

bullying, 135

burger joints: eating at food court, 132; healthier choices at, 125

Calf Stretch, 196p–97p

cardio exercise: golf as, 204–5; "kickin it" tunes for dancing, 190; Peachtree 5K Run/Walk Race, 9p, 157; SOS (Save Our Skin) 5K walk/run race, 157–58

chain restaurants, 126–27

Chalk Talks: Dad: How Parents Can Help with eating out, 133–34; Dad: How Parents Can Help with good nutrition, 105–6; Dad: How Parents Can Help with making decision to change, 40–42; Dad: How Parents Can Help with healthy eating, 84–85; Mom: What Parents Can Do to get helpful information, 57; Parents: Kids Need *You!*, 67. *See also* Greene, Brian (Dad); parents

change: the aha moment leading to, 31, 32, 38, 64; getting your parents involved with your, 68–69; how parents can help with decision to, 40–42; lessons learned during process of, 47–48; Mark's Story on making a, 150–51; reaching the decision to, 27–29, 31, 38–39; Sarah's Story on making a, 80. *See also* overweight kids

change strategies: Chalk Talks from My Parents: Kids Need *You!* on, 67; eating smaller meals more often, 59; family-centered

support, 40–42; getting your parents involved with your, 68–69; learning about healthy eating, 49–50

The Cheesesteak Story, 20–22

childhood obesity: due to other health problems, 58; emotions and, 56; heredity and, 55–56; how diet impacts, 55; how lifestyle impacts, 56, 58; physical inactivity and, 55. *See also* overweight kids

Chinese food court place, 131

Chinese restaurants, 127–28

choices: eating out as being all about, 115–24; how kids get heavy because of others', 14; making decision to change, 27–29, 31, 38–39; making good food, 55; on physical activity, 55

cholesterol levels, 66

Clockwork Drill, 152–53

Coach Z: "Be the tree" advice by, 16–17, 19; helping to create the first-quarter game plan, 43; introduction to, 5; on turning golf into cardio exercise, 204. *See also* Team Tiger coaches

Coach Z top tips: on flexibility activities, 192; on In-Out Ladder Drill, 154; on quickness activities, 160; on strength activities, 182; on Tiger Tail Drill, 141

Crabtree, Stephen: findings on childhood obesity lifestyle by, 56, 58; on hereditary tendency toward type 2 diabetes, 61; on human body joints, 60; introduction to,

23, 53; on overcoming barriers to exercise, 63; professional background of, 53; on why overweight children feel tired all the time, 58–59

Craighead, Linda: on eating every three to four hours, 78; Hunger Meter tool introduced by, 74–75; introduction to, 23–24, 72; on knowing when you are hungry, 71, 73–75, 76; professional background of, 72; working to improve Greene family's healthy lifestyle, 81–82

Crunches Drill, 178p–79p

Cuts Drill, 146–49p

Dance Central (active video game), 174

Danny, 214p

David's Story, 184–85

desserts, 123

diabetes, 60–61

diet: dangers of fasting, 61; determined by your parents, 55; feeling tired because of poor, 58–59; how it impacts your health, 55, 60; importance of eating breakfast, 59, 77; Sarah's Story on changing her, 80; taking steps to change your, 59; three-step strategy for healthy, 77–79. *See also* eating; meals

dieting: cycle of, 37; special dangers for kids, 61–63; why it isn't the answer, 49, 61

diner food court place, 132

doctors: getting answers from, 57; getting checkup before starting weight-loss programs, 58; "He'll grow out of it" advice by, 52–53, 67

Dodgeball (film), 159

Double Leg Forward and Backward Line Hops Drill, 162p–63p

Double Leg Side-to-Side Line Hops Drill, 164p–67p

downsizing portions, 118–19p, 121

The Dr. Oz Show, 10, 24, 72

eating: at the same time every day, 77–78; emotional, 56, 87–88; every three to four hours, 78–79; how parents can help with, 105–6; using Hunger Meter when, 74–75, 77, 79, 82–83, 84–87; learning about healthy, 49–50, 61–63; learning to grocery shop for healthy, 89–90; Sarah's Story on learning about healthy, 80. *See also* diet

eating out: as being all about choices, 115–24; danger of overeating when, 113–15; how parents can help when, 133–34. *See also* restaurants

eating out strategies: downsize portions, 118–19, 121; going LEAN, 116, 125, 126–27; looking for "bad words" on menus, 118; at mall food courts, 131–32; order things not on the menu, 116–18; rack up Tiger points, 121–23; for specific types of restaurants, 125–29; Tigerize a fast-food salad, 123–24

Emmett, 213

emotional eating, 56, 87–88

EnerZ wrap, 92–93p

English muffin with peanut butter, 94p

exercise: agility drills, 137–38, 142–58; cardio, 9p, 157–58, 190, 204–5; conditioning, 138–39; flexibility drills, 136, 191–206; making commitment to, 135–36; overcoming barriers to, 63–65; Peachtree Road Race, 9p, 157; quickness drills, 136, 159–74; strength drills, 136, 175–90; tips on stretching, 192. *See also* physical inactivity

families: first-quarter game plan for, 42–44; how diet is determined by, 55; how food becomes part of celebrating by, 27–28p, 32, 54, 71; how they can help you "Be the tree," 19; Team Tiger *Ohana* (family), 18, 19; as your secret weapon, 17–19. *See also* parents

fast foods: Atlanta Little League concession stands, 129–31; barbecue joints, 127; burger joints, 125; chain restaurants, 126–27; food court, 131–32; strategies for eating out at, 113–15; sub shops, 126

fast-food salads, 123–24

fasting, 61

fatigue: conditioning exercises to overcome, 138–39; due to lack of physical exercise, 59; due to poor diet, 58–59

fatty liver, 66

Finneran, Brian, 3

first-quarter game plan, 42–44

flexibility activities: Calf Stretch, 196p–97p; Chest/Shoulder Stretch, 194p–95p; Coach Z's top tips on, 192; Hamstring Stretch, 202p–3p; Hip Flexor Stretch, 198p–99p; importance of developing agility through, 136, 191–92; A Tiger Tale on yoga class for, 206; tips on stretching during, 192

Florence, Drayton, 3

Florida State University, 175

food control strategies: step 1: eat at the same times every day, 77–78; step 2: eat every three to four hours, 78–79; step 3: use the Hunger Meter every time you want to eat, 79

food courts, 131–32

foods: deciding how much we need, 94–95; deciding if they are "worth it or not," 81–82; feeling tired because of eating unhealthy, 58–59; grocery shopping for, 89–91, 106–12; how they become part of family celebrations, 27–28p, 32, 54, 71; using Hunger Meter to make decisions on, 74–75, 77, 79, 82–83, 84–87; learning to make good choices, 55; learning to recognize your hunger for, 71–77; selecting restaurant, 113–34; toss out the junk, 106; understanding that it is not the enemy, 61–63. *See also* meals; snacks

fries, 122

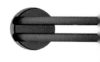

gallstones, 66

Georgia Dome: selected for first Team Tiger Camp, 11; welcoming kids to Team Tiger Camp, 5–8

glucose levels, 60–61

golf exercise, 204–5

Green Eagles [Green(e) Machine] football team: Alpharetta Youth Football All-Star game by, 209–16; Bulldozer Wedge play used by the, 35–36p, 193; the Cheesesteak Story on team chant of, 20–21; introduction to the, 20–21; photographs of the All-Star game of, 210p, 211p, 213p; photographs of the members of the, 214p, 215p. *See also* Alpharetta Youth Football All-Star game (2009)

Greene, Brian (Dad): Alpharetta Youth Football All-Star game coached by, 209–11; Alpharetta Youth Football All-Star game photo with Tiger and, 210p; The Cheesesteak Story role of, 20–22; deciding if food is "worth it or not," 81–82; in front of White House with Tiger, 39p; having a Man v. Food weekend with, 86–87; helping Tiger to reach decision to change, 31; response to "Be the tree" advice, 16; welcoming kids to Team Tiger Camp, 6. *See also* Chalk Talks

Greene family: celebrating with food by, 27–28p, 32, 54, 71; Chalk Talk on strategies adopted by, 40–42; first-quarter game plan by the, 42–44; helping to celebrate Tiger's name change, 27–28; learning to celebrate events and not the meal, 105–6; working to improve healthy lifestyle of, 81–82

Greene, Granni, 34, 71, 129–30

Greene, Kaila: asks Tiger if he would want to turn back time, 46; on being a Team Tiger member, 176; celebrating birthday of, 71; in fighting stance with Tiger, 52p; found in 90th percentile of height and weight, 52–53; introduction to, 8; weight loss by friend of, 25–26

Greene, Marsha (Mom): first-quarter game plan role of, 43; on 5K with Tiger, 64p, 157; on what parents can do to help, 57

Greene, Mike, 8

The Greene Room (restaurant private room), 37

Greene, Tiger: Alpharetta Youth Football All-Star game played by, 209–11; brother Zack and sister Kaila of, 7–8; *The Dr. Oz Show* appearance by, 10, 24; on founding of Team Tiger Foundation by, 8–9; retelling his journey in order to help others, 3–7; story of Tiger name, 33–34; why football plays such a big role in life of, 213–16. *See also* My journey; photographs

Greene, Zack: introduction to, 7–8; on learning about healthy eating, 130; next to very big pizza, 86p; photograph of Tiger with, 7p; Tiger playing basketball with, 69p

grocery shopping: going with Dad, 89–91; Shopping List! to copy for, 110–12; tips for parents on, 106, 108–9

Hamstring Stretch, 202*p*–3*p*

health problems: additional, 65–66; how knowledge can help you prevent, 68; how poor diet may result in, 55, 60; joint pain, 59–60; obesity as result of other, 58; Tiger's experience with, 38, 51–53; type 2 diabetes, 60–61. *See also* overweight kids

healthy eating. *See* eating

heart attack risk, 66

heart (grit or determination), 19

"He'll grow out of it" advice, 52–53, 67

hereditary: obesity and, 55–56; type 2 diabetes and, 61

high blood pressure, 66

high cholesterol, 66

Hip Flexor Stretch, 198*p*–99*p*

home-school academy, 43

hunger: emotional eating instead of genuine, 56, 87–88; learning to recognize your, 71, 73–75, 76; learning to recognize your stomach signals on, 76; three-step plan for controlling your, 77–79; two questions to ask yourself about, 73

Hunger Meter: getting to 4 and no more on the, 82–83; how parents can help you use the, 84–85; Hunger Meter magnet on refrigerator as reminder, 77; learning to use the, 75, 79; one of my 5 stories on using the, 85–87; Tiger's, 74

ice cream places, 132

In-Out Ladder Drill, 154*p*–56*p*

insulin, 60

Italian restaurants, 128

Japanese restaurants, 128

joint pain, 59–60

Jordan, Brian, 90*p*

junk foods, 106

Knopf, Dr., 56

Kozlowski, Brian, 3

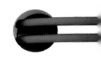

LEAN formula: applied to chain restaurants, 126–27; description of, 116; Tigerizing your eating out by going, 125

Leftwich, Byron, 3

lifestyle: changing your eating, 59; impact of inactive, 55; obesity relationship to, 56, 58; reaching the decision to change, 27–29, 31, 38–39, 40–42; working to improve your healthy, 81–82

Little League concession stands (Atlanta), 129–31

Madden NFL & NCAA Football (active video game), 174

Madden NFL (game), 12*p*

mall food courts, 131–32

Man v. Food (TV show), 85–86

Man v. Food weekend, 86*p*–87

Mark's Story, 150–51

Matt, 214

meals: breakfast, 59, 77, 92–94*p*; dinner, 99–102*p*; eating every three

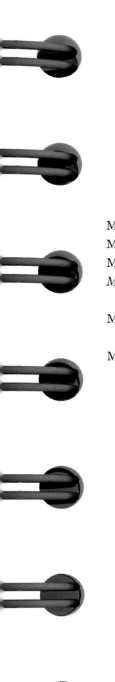

to four hours, 78–79; how they become part of family celebrations, 27–28p, 32, 54, 71; Hunger Meter used to plan for, 84–85; lunch, 95–98; restaurant, 113–34; serve water with, 106, 122; snacks, 7–79, 84–85, 103–4p; special occasion, 105. *See also* diet; foods

Melinda, Mrs., 43

Mexican restaurants, 128–29

Mikey, 214p

Motion Sports (active video game), 174

Muhammad Ali Line Shuffle Drill, 168p–69p

My journey: aha moment of, 31, 32, 38, 64; Alpharetta Youth Football All-Star game (2009) as closing chapter of, 209–16; cycle of dieting, weight gain, and health problem, 37–38; family support of, 40–44; following me in your own journey, 24–26; getting over my tunnel vision, 3–5; growing from chubby to "glob," 34–36; to help others begin their own journey, 1; learning to believe in yourself, 45–46; lessons learned from, 46–48; overcoming barriers to starting, 13–15; on reaching the decision to change, 27–29, 31, 38–39; writing letters to Nike and Atlanta Falcons, 43–44. *See also* Greene, Tiger; Your journey

nagging, 41

NFL Training Camp (active video game), 174

Nike, 43–44

North Carolina teachers, 30

Obama, Michelle, 39

Ohana (family), 18, 19

O'Houlihan, Patches, 159

overweight kids: ABCs of being a big kid, 65; able to follow in their own journey, 24–26; barriers to losing weight faced by, 13–15; "Be the tree" advice to, 16–17, 19; blaming by, 15; born to be big?, 54–56; dangers of fasting and diets for, 61–63; David's Story, 184–85; feeling tired all the time, 58–59; Find the Tiger in You! note to, 15; lack of choices allowed to, 14; learning to believe in yourself, 45–46; Mark's Story, 150–51; Sarah's Story, 80; secret weapons of, 17–19. *See also* change; childhood obesity; health problems

parents: A Note from Mrs. Kim to, 107–8; getting them involved with your change, 68–69; good nutrition tips for, 105–6; helping kids make decision to change, 40–42; helping kids when eating out, 133–34; Kids Need *You!*, 67; promoting healthy eating, 84–85. *See also* Chalk Talks; families

parent strategies: be generous with praise, 42; catch them doing well, 41; discuss your challenges openly, 42; don't nag—instead offer alternatives, 41; eating out

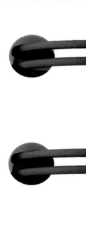

parent strategies *(continued)*
at restaurants, 133–34; to help gather information, 57; involve your children in the game plan, 41; let your child off the hook, 40; pledge your family's support, 40–41; promoting good nutrition, 105–6

Peachtree 5K Run/Walk Race (Atlanta), 9*p*, 157

Peterson, Mike, 3, 184

Philly Connection, 21

photographs: Alpharetta Youth Football All-Star game, 210*p*, 211*p*, 213*p*; Alpharetta Youth Football All-Star members, 214*p*, 215*p*; breakfast suggestions, 93*p*–94*p*; Bulldozer Wedge (football play), 36*p*; Calf Stretch, 196*p*–97*p*; celebrating legally changing name from Tyler to Tiger, 27–28*p*; Chest/Shoulder Stretch, 194*p*–95*p*; Crunches Drill, 178*p*–79*p*; cute picture of Tiger, 32*p*; Cuts Drill, 146–49*p*; Double Leg Forward and Backward Line Hops Drill, 162*p*–63*p*; Double Leg Side-to-Side Line Hops Drill, 164*p*–67*p*; downsizing portions, 119*p*; Hamstring Stretch, 202*p*–3*p*; Hip Flexor Stretch, 198*p*–99*p*; In-Out Ladder Drill, 154*p*–56*p*; Man v. Food weekend with Zack, 86*p*; Marcus Stroud and Tiger, 11*p*; Muhammad Ali Line Shuffle Drill, 168*p*–69*p*; the original Team Tiger, 18*p*; Planks Drill, 180*p*–81*p*; Push-Ups Drill, 188*p*–89*p*; Quad Stretch,

200*p*–201*p*; Squats Drill, 183*p*; T-Drill workout, 143*p*–45*p*; Tiger at the Breast Friends Golf Tournament (2009), 9*p*; Tiger with Atlanta Braves' Brian Jordan, 90*p*; Tiger at Team Tiger Camp, 25*p*; Tiger on a cruise, 14*p*; Tiger cuddling with puppy, 132*p*; Tiger and Dad at the Alpharetta Youth Football All-Star game, 210*p*; Tiger as Hulk, 83*p*; Tiger in fighting stance with Kaila, 52*p*; Tiger on 5K with mom, 64*p*; Tiger in front of the White House with dad, 39*p*; Tiger just before first 10K Peachtree Road Race, 9*p*; Tiger pitching a killer game, 114*p*; Tiger playing basketball with Zack, 69*p*; Tiger playing football, 22*p*, 45*p*; Tiger with Sakki (dog), 47*p*; Tiger's first touchdown (2011), 213*p*; Tiger showing off smarticles, 88*p*; Tiger and Zack, 7*p*; Triceps Dips Drill, 186*p*–87*p*; X-Hops Drill, 170*p*–71*p*. *See also* Greene, Tiger

physical inactivity: being overweight due to, 55; feeling tired due to, 59. *See also* exercise

physicians. *See* doctors

pizza delivery story, 32–33

pizza food court place, 131

Planks Drill, 180*p*–81*p*

playbook: description of, 23; Team Tiger's, 23–24

portion control, 118–19*p*, 121

Powerade Zero, 131

praise, 42

Push-Ups Drill, 188*p*–89*p*

Quad Stretch, 200p–201p

quickness activities: active video games, 174; Coach Z's top tips on, 160; Double Leg Forward and Backward Line Hops Drill, 162p–63p; Double Leg Side-to-Side Line Hops Drill, 164p–67p; importance of developing quickness through, 136, 159–61; Muhammad Ali Line Shuffle Drill, 168p–69p; Wall Reaction Drill, 172–73; X-Hops Drill, 170p–71p

Red Eagles, 35–36p

restaurants: barbecue joints, 127; burger joints, 125, 132; chain, 126–27; Chinese, 127–28, 131; giving a makeover to your favorite, 129–31; how parents can help when eating at, 133–34; Italian, 128; Japanese, 128; Mexican, 128–29; sub shops, 126. *See also* eating out

role models: deciding to become a, 15; needing a, 14

Sakki (dog), 47p

salad food court place, 132

salads: substituting fries for, 122; Tigerizing a fast-food, 123–24

Sarah's Story, 80

Scout (dog), 161

secret weapons: heart (grit or determination), 19; your family as a, 17–18; your Team Tiger family, 18

Shane's Rib Shack, 5, 117, 120

Shopping List!, 110–12

sleep apnea, 66

snacks: eating every three to four hours, 78–79; Hunger Meter used to plan for, 84–85; keeping up your energy with, 103–4p. *See also* foods

SOS (Save Our Skin) 5K walk/run race, 157–58

soy sausage links, 92–93p

special occasion meals: celebrating the event and not the, 105; how we overeat during, 27–28p, 32, 54, 71

Sports Illustrated, 161

Squats Drill, 182–83p

strength activities: Coach Z's Top Tips on, 182; Crunches Drill, 178p–79p; David's Story on, 184–85; importance of developing agility through, 136, 175, 177; Planks Drill, 180p–81p; Push-Ups Drill, 188p–89p; Squats Drill, 182–83p; Triceps Dips Drill, 186p–87p

stretching exercise, 192

stroke risk, 66

Stroud, Marcus: David's Story on meeting, 184; helping to organize first Team Tiger Camp, 10–12; helping to welcome new kids to Team Tiger Camp, 3, 6, 8; photographed with Tiger, 11p

sub shops, 126

Taco Mac, 115, 120

T-Drill, 142–45p

Team Tiger Camp: activity stations set up at the, 136; David's Story on attending, 184–85; having

Team Tiger Camp (*continued*)
restaurant owners speak to kids
at, 120; Mark's Story on attending,
150–51; the North Carolina
Teachers attending, 30; playbook of,
23–24; the story of the first, 10–12
Team Tiger Cheer, 20–22
Team Tiger coaches: Kim Wilson, 24,
91–95, 107–8; Linda Craighead,
23–24, 71–76, 78, 81–82; Shane
Thompson, 5, 24, 117, 185; Stephen
Crabtree, 23, 53, 56, 58–61. *See
also* Coach Z
Team Tiger Foundation: the original
Team Tiger, 18*p*; origins and
founding of, 8–9; welcoming the
new kids to, 5–8
Team Tiger healthier choice menu,
130–31
Team Tiger *Ohana* (family), 18, 19
Thompson, Shane: introduction to,
24, 117; professional background
of, 117; Team Tiger Camp
participation by, 185; welcoming
the kids to Team Tiger Camp, 5
Tiger points: blow off the bread
basket for, 122; choosing either
mayo or cheese, 123; description
of, 121; ditch dessert, 123;
drinking two glasses of water
with meal for, 122; learning to say
"on the side," 123; swap fries for
something green, 122
A Tiger's Tale: on being able to do
the Bulldozer Wedge, 193; on
conditioning exercise, 138–39;
having restaurant owners speak to
kids, 120; on yoga class, 206
Tiger Tail Drill, 140–41

Tiger Woods PGA Tour (active video
game), 174
Triceps Dips Drill, 186*p*–87*p*
triglyceride levels, 66
type 2 diabetes, 60–61

video games, 174

Wall Ball (game), 159–60
Wall Reaction Drill, 172–73
water drinking: during family meals
for everyone, 106; "Tiger points"
for two glasses with restaurant
meal, 122
Whole Food Market, 130
Wii Fit (active video game), 174
Wii Sports (active video game), 174
Wilson, Kim: on deciding how
much food we need, 94–95; on
importance of eating breakfast,
92–94*p*; introduction to, 24, 91–
92; a note to parents from, 107–8;
professional background of, 91
Woods, Tiger, 33, 34

X-Hops Drill, 170*p*–71*p*

yoga class, 206
Your journey: beginning the road to,
207; choosing to follow my own
journey with, 24–26. *See also* My
journey

Zumwalt, Andrew. *See* Coach Z

Scan this code with your smartphone to be linked to bonus materials for *SACKING OBESITY* and other healthy living books and information.

You can also text keyword TIGER to READIT (732348) to be sent a link to the mobile website.

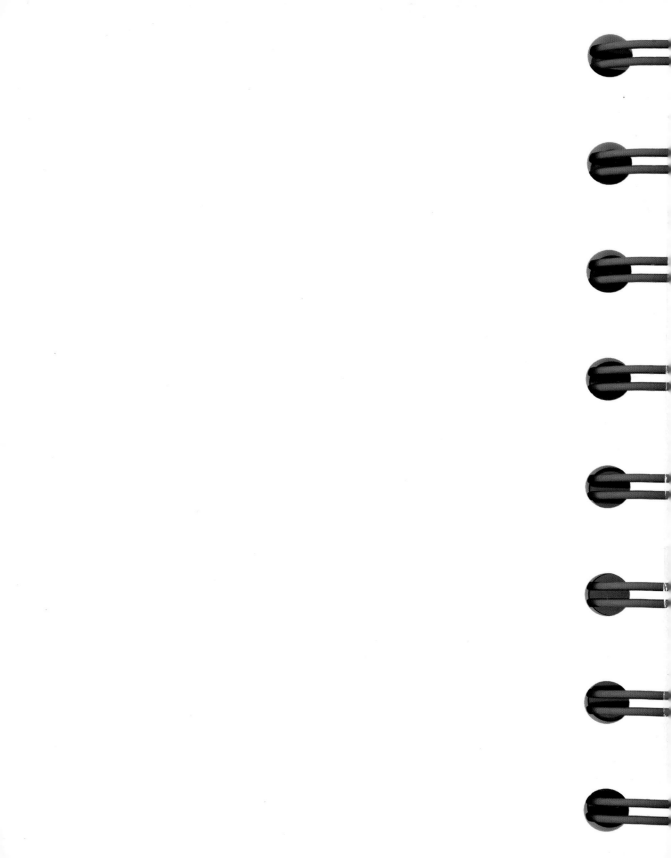